D1469495

Nutrition and Heart Disease

Volume I

Editor
Ronald R. Watson, Ph.D.
Research Professor
Department of Family and
Community Medicine
Health Sciences Center
University of Arizona
Tucson, Arizona

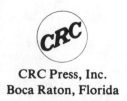

CRC Press, Inc.
Boca Raton, Florida

Library of Congress Cataloging-in-Publication Data
Nutrition and heart disease.

Includes bibliographies and index.
    1. Heart—Diseases—Nutritional aspects.
2. Heart—Diseases—Prevention. 3. Heart—
Diseases—Diet therapy.   I. Watson, Ronald R.
(Ronald Ross) [DNLM: 1. Cardiovascular Diseases—
diet therapy. 2. Cardiovascular Diseases—
prevention & control. 3. Diet—adverse effects.
4. Nutrition. WG 100 N976]
RC682.N87 1987   616.1′205   87-8070
ISBN 0-8493-4640-1 (set)
ISBN 0-8493-4641-X (v. 1)
ISBN 0-8943-4642-8 (v. 2)

    Direct all inquiries to CRC Press, Inc., 2000 Corporate Blvd., N.W., Boca Raton, Florida, 33431.

© 1987 by CRC Press, Inc.

International Standard Book Number 0-8493-4640-1 (set)
International Standard Book Number 0-8493-4641-X (v. 1)
International Standard Book Number 0-8493-4642-8 (v. 2)
Library of Congress Card Number 87-8070
Printed in the United States

PREFACE

Nutritional Needs of the Aging Adult

Nutritional needs for the aging adults are a special case! It is clear from the literature that in some areas many people believe the aging adult is just an extrapolation of, or maybe the same as the mature adult. While the aged adult may have somewhat reduced dietary intakes and metabolic rates, needs are otherwise very similar and may be identical to young adults. This may actually be the fact for some nutrients. On the other hand, it is clear that the tissue levels of some nutrients such as B6 change radically from childhood to mature adulthood and aging. These changes may be associated with the use of other nutrients including alcohol, smoking, and possibly with changed dietary habits, or altered absorption retention of the nutrient. However, these changes may reflect the needs of the adult and particularly the aging adult. Certainly one thing that the reviews included in these two volumes show, is that much information has been obtained and much more is needed to be obtained on the special cases and problems of the aging adult as distinguished from teenagers, children, pregnant women, and middle-aged adults. As our population ages and has a greater number of people in the aged category, it is critical to understand their specialized needs. In addition, it is important to understand that chronological aging is a combination of many factors. It is not just physiological changes of the body due to increasing longevity, it is also influenced by exercise, diet, disease, and sociological and psychological parameters. The aging adult is not a single individual in various decades of life, rather, they are a disparage group of individuals. Studies have really been lacking to distinguish between the particular reasons which cause individuals to age or change differently. These are important considerations in reviewing dietary needs and the effects that dietary intakes and problems have on the aging adult. It is not possible to routinely extrapolate from the studies of mature, healthy, young men and women and determine the optimum needs for treating disease states and preventing problems in aging adults in their sixth to tenth decade of life. Specialized studies must be designed for them and are sorely lacking. Nevertheless, there are major advances that have been made in understanding the nutritional problems particularly as they relate to heart cardiovascular disease in the aging adult. These have been summarized with special emphasis on nutrition in the two volumes of this book.

Ronald Ross Watson
August, 1987

THE EDITOR

Ronald R. Watson Ph.D., attended the University of Idaho, graduating from Brigham Young University in Provo, Utah with a degree in Chemistry in 1966. He completed his Ph.D. degree in 1971 in Biochemistry from Michigan State University. His post-doctoral schooling was completed at the Harvard School of Public Health in Nutrition and Microbiology, including a 2-year post-doctoral research experience in Immunology. He was an Assistant Professor of Immunology and did research at the University of Mississippi Medical Center in Jackson, Mississippi from 1973 to 1974. He was an Assistant Professor of Microbiology and Immunology at the Indiana University Medical School from 1974 to 1978. He was an Associate Professor at Purdue University in the Department of Food and Nutrition from 1978 to 1982. In 1982, he joined the faculty at the University of Arizona in the Department of Family and Community Medicine, Nutrition section. In 1987, he was promoted to Research Professor. In addition he has been a member of the International Center for Medical Research in the area of nutrition and immunology in Cali, Colombia and associated with the Nutrition Institute in Cario, Egypt.

His research interests have involved studying the immune function under nutritional stress including research with human subjects. His major research interest involves effects of dietary materials on disease resistance and immune functions. This includes understanding the effects of alcohol and drug abuse on immunosuppression associated with AIDs, the role of vitamin A, and beta carotene as modulators of skin cancer resistance and immune function in people and animals. He has published 150 research papers and review chapters.

Dr. Watson is a member of several national and international nutrition, immunology, and cancer societies.

CONTRIBUTORS

Alexander C. Arntzenius, M.D.
Professor emeritus
Den Haag, Netherlands

Martina A. Diolulu, Ph.D
Research Fellow
National Heart Lung Blood Institute
National Institutes of Health
Bethesda, Maryland

Miguel A. Guzmán-F, Ph.D.
Professor
Departments of Pathology and Biometry
Louisiana State University Medical
  School
New Orleans, Louisiana

Jerome L. Hojnacki, Ph.D.
Professor and Director
Lipid Research Laboratory
Department of Biological Sciences
University of Lowell
Lowell, Massachusetts

David Kritchevsky, Ph.D.
Wistar Institute of Anatomy and Biology
Philadelphia, Pennsylvania

Daan Kromhout, Ph.D.
Professor
Institute of Social Medicine
University of Leiden
Leiden, Netherlands

Fred A. Kummerow, Ph.D.
Professor
Department of Food Science
Burnsides Research Laboratory
University of Illinois
Urbana, Illinois

Kai Y. Lei, Ph.D.
Associate Professor
Department of Nutrition and Food
  Sciences
University of Arizona
Tucson, Arizona

Donald J. McNamara, Ph.D.
Professor
Department of Nutrition and Food
  Science
University of Arizona
Tucson, Arizona

Robert J. Nicolosi, Ph.D.
Department of Clinical Science
University of Lowell
Lowell, Massachusetts

H. L. "Sam" Queen, M.A.
Health Care Educator
Editor/Publisher *Heart Talk*
Queen and Company
Colorado Springs, Colorado

Terrance L. Smith, Ph.D.
Senior Food Scientist
Department of Food Science
University of Illinois
Urbana, Illinois

Jack P. Strong, M.D.
Boyd Professor and Head
Department of Pathology
Louisiana State University Medical
  Center
New Orleans, Louisiana

Ronald R. Watson, Ph.D.
Research Professor
Department of Family and Community
  Medicine
Health Sciences Center
University of Arizona
Tucson, Arizona

Karen K. Willcox, M.S.
Research Assistant
Nutrition and Food Science
University of Arizona
Tucson, Arizona

TABLE OF CONTENTS

Chapter 1

DIETARY FIBER IN CARDIOVASCULAR DISEASE

David Kritchevsky

TABLE OF CONTENTS

I. INTRODUCTION

Dietary fiber is generally defined as plant material that is resistant to the enzymes of the alimentary tract. Fiber comprises a number of substances of varying chemical structure and morphology. Chemically, the materials which we call fiber are, with one exception, carbohydrate in nature; the exception is lignin. Fiber, regarded in view of its botanical function, presents three components, namely, cellulose, the major fibrillar component of the plant cell wall; hemicellulose and pectins, which form the cell matrix; and lignin, which is an encrusting substance present in the mature cell wall. The definition of fiber has been extended to include plant gums and mucilages such as gum arabic or guar gum. Two excellent reviews of plant wall fiber structure and function are available.[1,2]

What may be regarded as the modern fiber era dates to a paper by Cleave[3] which attributed many of the modern degenerative diseases to consumption of refined flour and refined sugar. Burkitt and Trowell began to express similar views about 10 years later.[4-6] The paper which brought home the message in the U.S. appeared in 1974.[7] It pointed to eight disease conditions prevalent in the U.S. but missing in Africa and attributed them to lack of fiber in our diets. It is important to point out, however, that the fiber hypothesis is based on a dietary lifestyle and not on addition of specific substances to our usual diet.

The effect of any treatment on development and progression of atherosclerosis in animals can be assessed easily by performing an autopsy at the termination of a given study. In man, influence of treatment is judged by effects on levels of serum or plasma lipids or lipoprotein levels. Thus, it is possible to discuss fiber effects on experimental animals as a function of serum or liver lipids or actual atherosclerotic involvement of the aorta or coronary vessels. Studies in humans are, at present, limited to reports of changes of lipid or lipoprotein levels or ratios. Influences of fiber on apolipoprotein levels have been described in a few instances.

II. ANIMAL STUDIES

The rat is very resistant to simple dietary induction of atherosclerosis[8] but effects of fiber on serum or liver lipid levels can provide insights concerning the action of specific fibers. Wells and Ershoff[9] compared serum and liver cholesterol levels in rats fed a basal fiber-free diet (B), B plus 1% cholesterol (BD), or BD plus 5% citrus or apple pectin or pectic acid. As Table 1 shows, the various pectins inhibited the cholesterol-induced increase in liver cholesterol but the pectic acid did not. It is evident, then, that not all types of fiber will reduce liver accumulation of dietary cholesterol in rats. While pectin,[9-11] guar[11,12] or locust bean gums,[10] lignin,[12] and oat bran[13,14] will reduce liver cholesterol levels, agar,[15] cellulose,[16,17] and alginic acid[16] increase hepatic cholesterol levels. Cellulose[18] increases total body cholesterol as well. Chen and Anderson[13,19] found that addition of cholesterol and cholic acid to a basal rat diet decreased the ratio of high density lipoprotein (HDL) cholesterol:total cholesterol by 70 to 74%. The decrease in this ratio was partially reversed by guar gum, pectin, or oat bran but not by wheat bran.

Pectin will reduce plasma and liver cholesterol levels in cholesterol-fed guinea pigs.[20] Cellulose increases cholesterolemia in guinea pigs fed a cholesterol-free diet.[21]

Rabbits fed saturated fat as part of a semipurified diet exhibit hypercholesterolemia and atherosclerosis,[22,23] whereas, saturated fat has no hyperlipidemic effect when added to laboratory ration.[24,25] Since the major difference between the two diets was the type of fiber, it was reasonable to suggest that the difference in effects was due to

Table 1

INFLUENCE OF FIBER ON PLASMA AND LIVER
CHOLESTEROL IN RATS[a]

| | Plasma cholesterol (mg/dl) | Liver cholesterol (g/100 g) | |
Diet		Total	% Ester
Basal[b]	94 ± 3	2.0 ± 0.1	23.6
Basal + 1% cholesterol (BC)	131 ± 12	24.7 ± 1.3	86.6
BC + 5% citrus pectin	106 ± 3	11.4 ± 1.3	77.2
BC + 5% apple pectin	104 ± 4	8.2 ± 0.8	72.0
BC + 5% pectic acid	117 ± 6	24.8 ± 2.2	86.7

[a]   After Wells and Ershoff.[9]
[b]   61% Sucrose, 24% casein, 10% cottonseed oil, and 5% salt mix.

Table 2

EFFECT OF SPECIAL DIETS ON ATHEROSCLEROSIS IN
RABBITS[a]

Fiber (%)[b]	Fat (%)[c]	No.	Cholesterol (mg/dl ± SEM)	Atherosclerosis (1—4 scale)
Cellulose (15)	HCNO (14)	11/15	207 ± 36	0.85
Cellulose (15)	HCNO (12) CR (2)	12/15	249 ± 41	0.90
Stock R (85)	HCNO (14)	7/15	64 ± 9	0.40
Stock (86)	HCNO (12) CR (2)	14/15	35 ± 2	0.25

[a]   After Kritchevsky and Tepper.[27,28]
[b]   Stock R: residue after lipid extraction; stock: commercial ration.
[c]   HCNO: hydrogenated coconut oil; CR: fat extracted from stock diet.

the fiber.[26] Experiments using various types of fats and fiber[27-29] showed that both the type of dietary fat and the type of fiber influenced cholesterolemia and atherosclerosis (Tables 2 and 3). Howard et al.[30] found that dilution of an atherogenic diet with an equal amount of stock diet inhibited atherogenesis and reduced cholesterol levels by 67%. Rabbits fed a semipurified diet containing cellulose exhibit hypercholesterolemia and atherosclerosis. Replacing the cellulose by wheat straw does not affect cholesterolemia but reduces the severity of atherosclerosis and replacement by alfalfa reduces both parameters.[31]

Guar gum and carrageenan are hypocholesterolemic in cholesterol-fed chickens.[32] When chickens were fed 0.6% cholesterol and 3% cellulose or pectin, the latter resulted in lower plasma cholesterol levels and significantly reduced severity of aortic and coronary atherosclerosis.[33]

Neither wheat, rice, or soy bran affect cholesterolemia in cynomolgus monkeys fed low (0.07 to 0.99%) levels of cholesterol.[34] When Vervet monkeys were fed a semipurified diet containing saturated fat and 15% fiber, alfalfa, and wheat straw were found to be less cholesterolemic than cellulose, and wheat straw was less sudanophilic as well.[35] (Table 4)

Earliest studies relating to possible mechanisms of action of fiber suggested that it reduced bile acid turnover.[36,37] Rats fed pectin excrete more bile acid than those fed cellulose[38] and chickens fed pectin excrete more lipid and more cholesterol than those

Table 3

INFLUENCE OF DIETARY FIBER ON ATHEROSCLEROSIS IN RABBITS[a]

Fat (20%)	Fiber (19%)	Cholesterol (mg/dl ± SEM)	Atherosis (% ± SEM)
Corn oil	Wheat straw	23 ± 4	0.7 ± 0.6
Corn oil	Cellulose	61 ± 5	1.3 ± 0.3
Corn oil	Cellophane	71 ± 6	5.0 ± 0.7
Butter fat	Wheat straw	114 ± 12	13 ± 3
Butter fat	Cellulose	133 ± 10	21 ± 3
Butter fat	Cellophane	216 ± 14	38 ± 7
Butter fat	Cellophane-peat (14:5)	141 ± 12	11 ± 2

[a]   After Moore.[29]

Table 4

EFFECT OF FIBER ON LIPID LEVELS AND AORTIC SUDANOPHILIA IN VERVET MONKEYS[a]

	Alfalfa	Fiber[b] cellulose	Wheat straw
Serum lipids (mg/dl ± SEM)			
Cholesterol	153 ± 9	174 ± 14	167 ± 8
Triglyceride	219 ± 51	213 ± 17	176 ± 24
Liver lipids (mg/g ± SEM)			
Cholesterol	2.65 ± 0.16	3.01 ± 0.10	2.56 ± 0.18
% Ester	22.2	21.9	19.9
Triglycerides	2.70 ± 0.41	3.93 ± 1.10	3.35 ± 0.62
Aortic sudanophilia			
% ± SEM	4.1 ± 2.9	3.8 ± 1.5	1.5 ± 0.4

[a]   After Kritchevsky et al.[39]
[b]   Diet consisted of 40% sucrose, 25% casein, 14% coconut oil, 15% fiber, 5% salt mix, and 1% vitamin mix. Fed for 23 weeks; 6 monkeys per group.

fed cellulose.[33] Rabbits fed a semipurified diet accumulate more cholesterol (endogenous and exogenous) in their serum and liver and excrete less cholesterol and bile acids than those fed a commercial ration[39] (Table 5).

Dietary fiber may exert its hypocholesterolemic effects by decreasing cholesterol absorption[39-41] or by increasing bile acid excretion.[38] Fiber has been shown to bind bile acids[42-44] and other lipids[45] in vitro and may have a similar effect in vivo. Pectin,[46,47] hard red spring wheat,[48] and oat bran[49] have all been shown to increase bile acid excretion in man.

III. HUMAN STUDIES

The possible influence of fiber on coronary disease in man can only be related to its effects on serum lipid and lipoprotein levels which are, in turn, risk factors for development of atherosclerosis. A compilation of results from 20 publications shows that wheat bran has virtually no effect on human cholesterol levels.[50] Compilation of data on pectin, however, reveal that it is hypocholesterolemic.[50] Vegetarians ingest a high

Table 5
CHOLESTEROL DISTRIBUTION IN
RABBITS FED COMMERCIAL OR
SEMIPURIFIED DIETS[a]

	Diet	
	Semipurified[b]	Commercial
Number	9/10	5/5
Serum lipids (mg/dℓ)		
Cholesterol	215 ± 17	93 ± 5
Triglyceride	131 ± 24	76 ± 24
Average atherosclerosis	1.35	0
Recovery of radioactivity[c]		
Serum		
^{3}H (dpm × 10^5)	4.03 ± 0.36	0.38 ± 0.11
^{14}C (dpm)	2757	ND[d]
Liver		
^{3}H (dpm × 10^6)	4.41 ± 0.52	1.34 ± 0.44
^{14}C (dpm × 10^4)	3.99 ± 0.59	1.05 ± 0.28
Aorta		
^{3}H	2160	920
^{14}C	198	88
Feces		
^{3}H (dpm × 10^6)	4.70 ± 1.5	19.0 ± 10.5
^{14}C (dpm × 10^3)	8.86 ± 1.6	11.2 ± 4.3

[a]   After Kritchevsky et al.[39]
[b]   Diet contained 40% carbohydrate, 25% casein, 14% co-
    conut oil, and 15% cellulose; fed for 6 months.
[c]   [1,2-^{3}H] cholesterol and [2-^{14}C] mevalonic acid injected
    intraperitoneally 72 hr before termination. ^{3}H = exoge-
    nous cholesterol; ^{14}C = endogenous cholesterol.
[d]   ND: not detectable.

fiber diet and they have been shown to have lower cholesterol and lipoprotein levels.[51-53] Sacks et al.[52] examined lipid levels in matched groups of macrobiotic vegetarians and controls and found the former to have significantly lower total plasma cholesterol and HDL cholesterol levels (Table 6). Knuiman and West[54] assayed total cholesterol and HDL cholesterol levels in omnivores, semi-lacto-ovo vegetarians, lacto-ovo vegetarians, and subjects on a macrobiotic regimen. Total cholesterol (mg/dℓ) and HDL cholesterol:total cholesterol ratios for the four groups were 212 ± 39 and 0.23 ± 0.07; 189 ± 39 and 0.28 ± 0.08; 181 ± 35 and 0.30 ± 0.08; and 147 ± 31 and 0.31 ± 0.08. A recent study in which lipids levels in Seventh Day Adventists were compared with fiber intake[55] showed that true vegetarians had the lowest serum cholesterol and highest serum triglyceride levels. Fiber intakes in the four groups were similar except for pectin which was more prominent in the diets of true vegetarians (Table 7). Pectin feeding (12 g/day) has been shown to decrease plasma low density lipoprotein (LDL) cholesterol levels by 18%[56] and guar-containing crispbread (13 g/day) has been found to reduce LDL cholesterol levels.[57] Oat bran decreased total serum cholesterol levels by 13% and LDL cholesterol levels by 14% while HDL cholesterol levels were unchanged.[49]

Stasse-Wothuis et al.[58] fed human volunteers diets high and low in fiber and high and low in cholesterol for 6 weeks. A diet high in fiber and cholesterol led to a 5% increase in serum total cholesterol and a 7% increase in HDL cholesterol. On a high fiber, low cholesterol diet, total and HDL cholesterol fell by 10 and 6%, respectively.

Table 6
PLASMA LIPIDS OF VEGETARIANS[a]

	Group	
	Vegetarian	Controls
Number	115	115
Cholesterol (mg/d*l* ± SEM)		
Total	126 ± 3	184 ± 3
VLDL	12 ± 0.7	17 ± 1
LDL	73 ± 2	118 ± 3
HDL	43 ± 1	49 ± 1
HDL/total	0.34	0.27
Triglycerides (mg/d*l* ± SEM)	59 ± 3	86 ± 4

[a] After Sacks et al.[52]

Table 7
SERUM LIPIDS AND DIETARY FIBER INTAKE IN MAN[a]

	Group[b]			
	V-SDA	LO-SDA	NV-SDA	GP
Number	18	25	25	22
Serum lipids (mg/d*l* ± SEM)				
Cholesterol	149 ± 8	192 ± 7	207 ± 7	214 ± 7
% HDL	24.4 ± 2.0	24.3 ± 1.6	21.8 ± 1.6	25.7 ± 1.8
Triglycerides	174 ± 17	142 ± 14	138 ± 14	97 ± 5
Fiber intake (g/kcal/day)				
NDF	14.5 ± 2.5	15.0 ± 1.0	13.5 ± 1.0	13.0 ± 1.0
Cellulose	2.5 ± 0.3	2.0 ± 0.2	1.5 ± 0.1	2.0 ± 0.2
Hemicellulose	11.0 ± 2.5	11.5 ± 1.0	11.0 ± 1.0	10.4 ± 1.0
Pectin	7.5 ± 1.0	4.5 ± 0.3	4.0 ± 0.3	4.0 ± 0.3
Lignin	0.8 ± 0.2	0.7 ± 0.2	0.5 ± 0.1	0.4 ± 0.1

[a] After Kritchevsky et al.[55]
[b] V-SDA: Vegetarian Seventh Day Adventists; LO-SDA: lacto-ovo vegetarian Seventh Day Adventists; NV-SDA: non-vegetarian Seventh Day Adventists; GP: general public.

When the diets contained low levels of fiber, the high cholesterol regimen resulted in a 4% increase in serum cholesterol and the low cholesterol diet led to a 7% decrease. The amount of cholesterol in the diet appears to have been the determining factor regardless of dietary fiber content.

Stasse-Wolthius et al.[59] also fed young subjects diets high in vegetables and fruits, citrus pectin, or bran. In the course of the 5-week study, cholesterol levels (mg/d*l*) in the control groups rose from 167 to 171; those in the vegetable/fruit group fell from 161 to 155; citrus pectin resulted in a reduction of serum cholesterol from 170 to 157; and the bran-fed subjects actually showed an increase from 165 to 178. Changes in ratio of HDL cholesterol:total cholesterol in the four groups were −2, 5, 10, and −3%, respectively. The group which exhibited the greatest reduction in serum cholesterol displayed the lowest increase in fecal weight (11 vs. 55% and 87% in vegetable/fruit and bran groups, respectively). Excretion of neutral steroids was increased significantly in the male subjects fed vegetable/fruit or citrus pectin and fecal excretion of bile acids was increased significantly in male subjects fed citrus pectin and decreased in those fed bran. In the female subjects, fecal excretion of neutral steroids and bile acids was increased significantly only in the group whose diet included bran.

The foregoing summary indicates that certain types of dietary fiber are hypocholesterolemic and hypolipoproteinemic in man. The effect is usually observed in the very low density lipoprotein (VLDL) and LDL fractions of the plasma. The mode of action of these substances has not been elucidated nor do we know which particular facets of fiber structure are responsible for the observed effects.

Burr and Sweetnam[60] had occasion to examine dietary and mortality records in Wales. They found that a vegetarian lifestyle was correlated with reduction of incidence of ischemic heart disease but fiber intake was not. These data reinforce the observations that it is a dietary lifestyle which includes high intake of vegetables and fruits which may lead to lower serum lipid levels and reduced risk of coronary disease.

REFERENCES

1. Kay, R. M., Dietary fiber, *J. Lipid Res.*, 23, 221, 1982.
2. Selvendran, R. R., The plant cell wall as a source of dietary fiber: chemistry and structure, *Am. J. Clin. Nutr.*, 39, 320, 1984.
3. Cleave, T. L., The neglect of natural principles in current medical practice, *J. R. Nav. Med. Serv.*, 42, 55, 1956.
4. Burkitt, D. P., Related disease - related cause, *Lancet*, 2, 1229, 1969.
5. Trowell, H., Crude dietary fibre and atherosclerosis, *Atherosclerosis*, 16, 138, 1972.
6. Trowell, H., Coronary heart disease and dietary fiber, *Am. J. Clin. Nutr.*, 28, 798, 1975.
7. Burkitt, D. P., Walker, A. R. P., and Painter, N. S., Dietary fiber and disease, *JAMA*, 229, 1068, 1974.
8. Kritchevsky, D., Animal models for atherosclerosis research, in *Hypolipidemic Agents*, Kritchevsky, D., Ed., Springer Verlag, Berlin, 1975, 216.
9. Wells, A. F. and Ershoff, B. H., Beneficial effects of pectin in prevention of hypercholesterolemia and increase in liver cholesterol in cholesterol-fed rats, *J. Nutr.*, 74, 87, 1961.
10. Ershoff, B. H. and Wells, A. F., Effects of guar gum, locust bean gum and carrageenan on liver cholesterol of cholesterol-fed rats, *Proc. Soc. Exp. Biol. Med.*, 11, 580, 1962.
11. Koo, S. I. and Stanton, P., Effects of cellulose, pectin and guar gum on the distribution of serum cholesterol among lipoprotein fractions, *Nutr. Rep. Int.*, 24, 395, 1981.
12. Story, J. A., Baldino, A., Czarnecki, S. K., and Kritchevsky, D., Modification of liver cholesterol accumulation by dietary fiber in rats, *Nutr. Rep. Int.*, 25, 783, 1982.
13. Chen, W. J. L. and Anderson, J. W., Effects of plant fiber in decreasing total cholesterol and increasing high density lipoprotein cholesterol, *Proc. Soc. Exp. Biol. Med.*, 162, 310, 1979.
14. Chen, W. J. L., Anderson, J., and Gould, M. R., Effects of oat bran, oat gum and pectin on lipid metabolism of cholesterol-fed rats, *Nutr. Rep. Int.*, 24, 1093, 1981.
15. Tsai, A. C., Elias, J., Keeley, J. J., Lin, R. S. C., and Robson, J. R. K., Influence of certain dietary fibers on serum and tissue cholesterol levels in rats, *J. Nutr.*, 106, 118, 1976.
16. Kiriyama, S., Okazaki, Y., and Yoshida, A., Hypocholesterolemic effect of polysaccharides and polysaccharide-rich foodstuffs in cholesterol-fed rats, *J. Nutr.*, 97, 382, 1969.
17. Kritchevsky, D., Ryder, E., Fishman, A., Kaplan, M., and DeHoff, J. L., Influence of dietary fiber on food intake, feed efficiency and lipids in rats, *Nutr. Rep. Int.*, 25, 783, 1982.
18. Mueller, M. A., Cleary, M. P., and Kritchevsky, D., Influence of dietary fiber on lipid metabolism in meal-fed rats, *J. Nutr.*, 113, 2229, 1983.
19. Chen, W. L. and Anderson, J. W., Effects of guar gum and wheat bran on lipid metabolism in rats, *J. Nutr.*, 109, 1028, 1962.
20. Wells, A. F. and Ershoff, B. H., Comparative effects of pectin NF administration on the cholesterol-fed rabbit, guinea pig, hamster and rat, *Proc. Soc. Exp. Biol. Med.*, 111, 147, 1962.
21. Riccardi, B. A. and Fahrenbach, M. J., Effect of guar gum and pectin NF on serum and liver lipids of cholesterol-fed rats, *Proc. Soc. Exp. Biol. Med.*, 124, 749, 1967.
22. Lambert, G. F., Miller, J. P., Olsen, R. T., and Frost, D. V., Hypercholesterolemia and atherosclerosis induced in rabbits by purified high fat rations devoid of cholesterol, *Proc. Soc. Exp. Biol. Med.*, 97, 544, 1958.
23. Malmros, H. and Wigand, G., Atherosclerosis and defiency of essential fatty acids, *Lancet*, 2, 749, 1959.

24. Kritchevsky, D., Moyer, A. W., Tesar, W. C., Logan, J. B., Brown, R. A., Davies, M. C., and Cox, H. R., Effect of cholesterol vehicle in experimental atherosclerosis, *Am. J. Physiol.*, 178, 30, 1954.

25. Kritchevsky, D. and Tepper, S. A., Cholesterol vehicle in experimental atherosclerosis. VI. Long-term effects of fats and fatty acids in a cholesterol-free diet, *J. Atheroscler. Res.*, 4, 113, 1964.

26. Kritchevsky, D., Experimental atherosclerosis in rabbits fed cholesterol-free diets, *J. Atheroscler. Res.*, 4, 103, 1964.

27. Kritchevsky, D. and Tepper, S. A., Factors affecting atherosclerosis in rabbits fed cholesterol-free diets, *Life Sci.*, 4, 1467, 1965.

28. Kritchevsky, D. and Tepper, S. A., Experimental atherosclerosis in rabbits fed cholesterol-free diets: influence of chow components, *J. Atheroscler. Res.*, 8, 357, 1968.

29. Moore, J. H., The effect of the type of roughage in the diet on plasma cholesterol levels and aortic atherosis in rabbits, *Br. J. Nutr.*, 21, 207, 1967.

30. Howard, A. N., Gresham, G. A., Jennings, I. W., and Jones, D., The effect of drugs on hypercholesterolaemia and atherosclerosis induced by semisynthetic, low cholesterol diets, *Prog. Biochem. Pharamacol.*, 2, 117, 1967.

31. Kritchevsky, D., Tepper, S. A., Williams, D. E., and Story, J. A., Experimental atherosclerosis in rabbits fed cholesterol-free diets. VII. Interaction of animal and vegetable protein with fiber, *Atherosclerosis*, 26, 397, 1977.

32. Fahrenbach, M. J., Riccardi, B. A. and Grant, W. C., Hypocholesterolemic activity of mucilaginous polysaccharides in white leghorn cockerels, *Proc. Soc. Exp. Biol. Med.*, 123, 321, 1966.

33. Fisher, H., Soller, W. G., and Griminger, P., The retardation by pectin of cholesterol-induced atherosclerosis in the fowl, *J. Atheroscler. Res.*, 6, 292, 1966.

34. Malinow, M. R., McLaughlin, P., Papworth, L., Naito, H. K., and Lewis, L. A., Effect of bran and cholestyramine on plasma lipids in monkeys, *Am. J. Clin. Nutr.*, 29, 905, 1976.

35. Kritchevsky, D., Davidson, L. M., Krendel, D. A., Van der Watt, J. J., Russell, D., Friedland, S., and Mendelsohn, D., Influence of dietary fiber on aortic sudanophilia in vervet monkeys, *Ann. Nutr. Metab.*, 25, 125, 1981.

36. Portman, O. W. and Murphy, P., Excretion of bile acids and hydroxysterols by rats, *Arch. Biochem. Biophys.*, 76, 367, 1958.

37. Portman, O. W., Nutritional influences on the metabolism of bile acids, *Am. J. Clin. Nutr.*, 8, 462, 1960.

38. Leveille, G. A. and Sauberlich, H. E., Mechanisms of the cholesterol-depressing effect of pectin in the cholesterol-fed rat, *J. Nutr.*, 88, 209, 1966.

39. Kritchevsky, D., Tepper, S. A., Kim, H. K., Moses, D. E., and Story, J. A., Experimental atherosclerosis in rabbits fed cholesterol-free diets. IV. Investigation into the source of cholesterolemia, *Exp. Mol. Pathol.*, 22, 11, 1977.

40. Hyun, S. A., Vahouny, G. V., and Treadwell, C. R., Effect of hypocholesterolemic agents on intestinal cholesterol absorption, *Proc. Soc. Exp. Biol. Med.*, 112, 496, 1963.

41. Vahouny, G. V., Roy, T., Gallo, L. L., Story, J. A., Kritchevsky, D., Cassidy, M., Grund, B. M., and Treadwell, C. R., Dietary fiber and lymphatic absorption of cholesterol in the rat, *Am. J. Clin. Nutr.*, 31, 5208, 1978.

42. Eastwood, M. A. and Hamilton, D., Studies on the adsorption of bile salts to non-absorbed components of the diet, *Biochim. Biophys. Acta*, 152, 165, 1968.

43. Kritchevsky, D. and Story, J. A., Binding of bile salts *in vitro* by nonnutritive fiber, *J. Nutr.*, 104, 458, 1974.

44. Story, J. A. and Kritchevsky, D., Comparison of the binding of various bile acids and bile salts *in vitro* by several types of fiber, *J. Nutr.*, 106, 1292, 1976.

45. Vahouny, G. V., Tombes, R., Cassidy, M. M., Kritchevsky, D., and Gallo, L. L., Dietary fibers. V. Binding of bile salts, phospholipids and cholesterol from mixed micelles by bile acid sequestrants and dietary fibers, *Lipids*, 15, 102, 1980.

46. Kay, R. M. and Truswell, A. S., Effect of citrus pectin on blood lipids and fecal steroid excretion in man, *Am. J. Clin. Nutr.*, 30, 171, 1977.

47. Miettinen, T. A. and Tarpila, S., Effect of pectin on serum cholesterol, fecal bile acids and biliary lipids in normolipidemic and hyperlipidemic individuals, *Clin. Chim. Acta*, 79, 471, 1977.

48. Spiller, G. A., Wong, L. G., Nunes, J. D., Story, J. A., Petro, M. S., Furumoto, E. J., Alton-Spiller, M., Whittam, J. H., and Scala, J., Effect of four levels of hard wheat bran on fecal composition and transit time in healthy young women, *Fed. Proc. Fed. Am. Soc. Exp. Biol.*, 43, 392, 1984.

49. Kirby, R. W., Anderson, J. W., Sieling, B., Rees, E. D., Chen, W. J. L., Miller, R. E., and Kay, R. M., Oat bran intake selectively lowers serum low density lipoprotein cholesterol concentrations of hypercholesterolemic men, *Am. J. Clin. Nutr.*, 34, 824, 1981.

50. Kay, R. M. and Truswell, A. S., Dietary fiber: effects on plasma and bilary lipids in man, in *Medical Aspects of Dietary Fiber*, Spiller, G. A. and Kay, R. M., Eds., Plenum Press, New York, 1980, 153.

51. Hardinge, M. G. and Stare, F. J., Nutritional studies of vegetarians. II. Diet and serum levels of cholesterol, *Am. J. Clin. Nutr.,* 2, 83, 1954.
52. Sacks, F. M., Castelli, W. P., Donner, A., and Kass, E. H., Plasma lipids and lipoproteins in vegetarians and controls, *N. Engl. J. Med.,* 292, 1148, 1975.
53. Burselm, J., Schonfeld, G., Howard, M. A., Werdman, S. W., and Miller, J. P., Plasma apoprotein and lipoprotein lipids levels in vegetarians, *Metabolism,* 27, 711, 1978.
54. Knuiman, J. T. and West, C. E., The concentration of cholesterol in serum and in various lipoproteins in macrobiotic, vegetarian and non-vegetarian men and boys, *Atherosclerosis,* 43, 71, 1982.
55. Kritchevsky, D., Tepper, S. A., and Goodman, G., Diet, nutrition intake, and metabolism in populations at high and low risk for colon cancer. Relationship of diet to serum lipids, *Am. J. Clin. Nutr.,* 40, 921, 1984.
56. Durrington, P. N., Manning, A. P., Bolton, C. H., and Hartog, M., Effect of pectin on serum lipids and lipoproteins, whole gut transit time and stool weight, *Lancet,* 2, 394, 1976.
57. Jenkins, D. J. A., Reynolds, D., Slavin, B., Leeds, A. R., Jenkins, A. L., and Jepson, E. M., Dietary fiber and blood lipids: treatment of hypercholesterolemia with guar crispbread, *Am. J. Clin. Nutr.,* 33, 575, 1980.
58. Stasse-Wolthius, M., Hautvast, J. G. A. J., Hermus, R. J. J., Katan, M. B., Bausch, J. E., Reitberg-Brussnard, J. H., Velma, J. P., Zondervan, J. E., Eastwood, M. A., and Brydon, G. R., The effect of a natural high fiber diet on serum lipids, fecal lipids and colonic function, *Am. J. Clin. Nutr.,* 32, 1881, 1979.
59. Stasse-Wolthius, M., Alberts, H. F. F., Van Jeveren, J. G. C., Wil de Jong, J., Hautvast, J. G. A. J., Hermus, R. J. J., Katan, M. B., Brydon, G. B., and Eastwood, M. A., Influence of dietary fiber from vegetables and fruits, bran or citrus pectin on serum lipids, fecal lipids and colonic function, *Am. J. Clin. Nutr.,* 33, 1745, 1980.
60. Burr, M. L. and Sweetnam, P. M., Vegetarianism, dietary fiber and mortality, *Am. J. Clin. Nutr.,* 36, 873, 1982.

Chapter 2

DIET AS A POTENT MODIFIER OF CARDIOVASCULAR RISK: HAS SOMETHING BEEN OVERLOOKED?

H. L. "Sam" Queen

TABLE OF CONTENTS

I. THE DIET-HEART VIEWPOINT: IT MAY BE TOO SIMPLISTIC

There is today general acceptance that the risk for heart disease increases as total serum cholesterol (TSC) rises above the norm. What has been lacking, until recently, is solid evidence that a reduction in TSC actually reduces heart risk. The "proof" was provided by the analysis of data from the popular Lipid Research Clinic (LRC) Study,[1] an extensive 7½-year program, and the most expensive ($150 million) heart disease research project ever undertaken. The authors' contention that an elevated TSC is an important risk factor received little criticism, but much dissention has since emerged, directed toward the premise that "an elevated TSC is THE major cause of heart attack". Conservative scientists[2-3] believe that an asterisk (*) should be added to this statement and to the following summation: People with an elevated TSC can expect to lessen their heart risk through lowering TSC*; that success can be attained through either lifestyle changes, or through combining lifestyle with a cholesterol-lowering drug*; and that the lifestyle regimen should emphasize the low-fat/low-cholesterol diet as prescribed for the LRC participants*. The message in this chapter is to explain the need for the proposed asterisk, that the simplistic approach as now recommended may be just that — too simplistic for optimal health and prevention of premature death due to all causes.

A. The Underlying Cause Hypothesis

While the present diet/heart prescription does appear prudent, there are many unanswered questions and potential pitfalls. Beyond age 55, for instance, the health risk of an elevated TSC steadily declines. The reason for this is not completely understood, but genetics may play a protective as well as a causal role. "It has been calculated," said Dr. Michael F. Oliver, The Duke of Edinburgh Professor of Cardiology, The University of Edinburgh, Edinburgh, Scotland, "that between 40 and 45% of any individual serum cholesterol concentration is genetically determined." This, he believes, may be the most important "underlying factor" and, of course, it is immutable, which makes one question the wisdom during the latter years of limiting cholesterol and fat. In addition, the aging process brings certain limitations in the selection of food, which makes it important to the health of many elderly people that foods with high nutritional density, such as eggs, not be forbidden. It is often wrongly assumed by these people, because of the publicity given cholesterol, that an elevated TSC is the direct result of excess fat and cholesterol in the diet. The common misconception is that a certain number of grams of fat and cholesterol in the diet translate to an equivalent rise in blood cholesterol. It is far more correct to state that the over-consumption of fat and cholesterol is likely to be consistent with a lifestyle of many unhealthy practices that, with or without genetic influence, lead to an elevated TSC. There may be underlying factors in that lifestyle that are far more important to the outcome than the quantity of fat and cholesterol. Dr. E. H. Ahrens, Jr., of Rockefeller University believes there are other important considerations that may be felt for years to come.

"Looking into the future," said Dr. Ahrens, "there is a danger that many young researchers will concede early on that the diet-heart question has been solved." Dr. Ahrens' reckoning can be justified by the broad support given the current diet-heart viewpoint by the popular lay press and mass media. This effective campaign has injuriously suppressed the view that an elevated TSC has an underlying cause. The underlying cause hypothesis, accepted as fact, would otherwise mean that an elevated TSC must be interpreted as a symptom rather than as a cause of heart disease. And, admittedly, while the symptom itself may promote atherosclerosis and thereby justify the present diet-heart viewpoint, there remains the danger that the regimen now employed for lowering cholesterol may not address the underlying defect(s). Rather, the regimen may mask the major symptoms by reducing TSC and perhaps other blood lipids without solving the basic problem. If this should occur, atherosclerosis may continue quietly and undetected, or the defect may manifest later as another disease. In yet another possible scenario, the cholesterol-lowering regimen may interact with the underlying defect in a negative and unhealthy manner. Any one of these possibilities, or a combination thereof, may have been the reality for those few people in the LRC Study who experienced a lower TSC but who died anyway.

It should be stated that within the test group in the LRC Study, as compared to the control group, there was a significant reduction in heart deaths. Yet, when total deaths are compared, there is no statistical difference between the two groups. The reduction in heart deaths in the study group was accompanied by an increase in deaths due to other, unexpected causes that have not been satisfactorily explained. This is important but not unusual. There is a paper to be published in the *Lancet* which reviews the combined results of 16 long-term clinical trials, indicating that the extent to which there has been a reduction in cardiovascular deaths is precisely offset by the increase in noncardiovascular deaths.

In retrospect, within the LRC Study, there may have been some pecularity about the mysterious underlying cause that made the low-fat/low-cholesterol diet correct for those individuals who lived to complete the study, but ineffective and perhaps even harmful to those who unexpectedly and prematurely died of heart disease and other causes. "The problem," said Dr. Oliver, "is that many health promoters seem to be unable to distinguish between reduction of risk and reduction of coronary heart disease (CHD). These are not the same." "Furthermore," Dr. Oliver argues, "it does not impress me greatly to read the results of expensive and lengthy trials which show that serum cholesterol (or LDL cholesterol) concentrations have been reduced but CHD has remained unchanged." This, he believes, is why it is important to continue researching cholesterol and to have the flexibility to insert into the diet-heart perspective whatever changes are appropriate. To do so, however, will require the fullest cooperation of the media. Can giant publications such as *Time* magazine, for instance, show this same flexibility? Can they maintain the openness that is needed to question the accuracy of their own reporting, especially after touting a particular viewpoint? If not, then any new findings that require change may be difficult and awkward to implement. Disregarding this possible restraint and professional embarrassment, there remains the potential for many underlying causes of heart disease, many of which are discussed in the various chapters of this book. The discussion here, while nonetheless significant, is limited to only two of these possibilities — the effect of excesses of estrogen and insulin.

II. HEART DISEASE AND EXCESS INSULIN

In 1976, Robert V. Fischer of Des Moines, Iowa, then an investigative writer and editor who was teamed with this investigative writer, reasoned the following: since advanced arterial disease is a feature of treated diabetes perhaps insulin plays a causal role in atherosclerosis. Earlier reports on animals seemed to agree. Arterial lesions increased in both diabetic and nondiabetic test animals in proportion to the quantity of insulin administered.[4-8] Together, we looked at reports of patients who had heart attacks. Sorge[9] reported that the incidence of myocardial infarction increases as the fasting level of plasma insulin increases. His findings were consistent with the earlier work of Kashyap,[10] who reported that both asymptomatic diabetics and nondiabetic atherosclerotic subjects had a higher plasma insulin when fasting than did healthy people. The association that linked insulin with heart disease had by then received our full attention, which prompted a call to the diabetes branch of the National Institutes of Health (NIH). An NIH spokesman pointed to the work of Harrison,[11] who just reported that insulin resistance and an elevated fasting insulin (not insulin deficiency) was positively associated with arterial disease. Shortly thereafter, Epstein and Stout[12] published supporting evidence that encouraged a look at population studies. Both researchers suggested that a high plasma insulin might be an underlying factor in arterial disease and heart attack.

A. Population Studies

From 1978 to 1979 there were three major population studies plus an important prospective study that confirmed Mr. Fischer's original suspicion. The Paris Prospective Study[13] demonstrated that heart risk was directly proportional to the fasting level of plasma insulin. Even the smallest rise in insulin increased heart risk in these people. And, when an elevated insulin was combined with low blood sugar, the risk increased 4.6-fold. Logan and Oliver,[14] during the same year, compared insulin and TSC as risk factors among Stockholm and Edinburgh men. While the incidence of heart disease was much greater in one country than in the other, the average TSC in men from either country was about equal. TSC, the researchers determined, was not a satisfactory determinant of obstructive arterial disease. Serum insulin, however, was an excellent predictor of a heart attack. It was consistently higher in men from the locale where the incidence of heart disease was the greatest.

Pyorala,[15] in 1979, compared the results from two population studies in Finland — the Helsinki Policeman Study and the Social Insurance Institutions (SII) Coronary Heart Disease Study. He studied the relationship of the insulin response to glucose feeding to the incidence of CHD. Pyorala's finding served as mortar to pull together the Fischer hypothesis. He observed that while blood sugar is not an independent predictor and certainly not the cause of heart disease in diabetes, an exaggerated insulin response to a high carbohydrate meal is a strong predictor and a major underlying cause of heart disease — acting independently of diagnosed diabetes and other risk factors.

In 1975, reporting on patients who would later develop diabetes,[16] Dr. Joseph Kraft learned that an elevated basal insulin and an exaggerated insulin response 1 hr and longer following a high carbohydrate meal was the earliest *in situ* predictor of diabetes. And, in cases where an excess of insulin is the underlying problem, this same criterion translates to the earliest event in the onset of arterial disease.

The Brusselton Study Results helped to clarify the insulin role further. Wellborn[17] et al., reported that the association of insulin with heart disease is consistent in men, but not in women. This is not surprising, however, since there is known to be a sex-linked difference in insulin sensitivity relative to the type and location of adipose tissue.[18] The evidence suggests that sex hormones play a key role in potentiating male atherosclerosis. Before looking further into this possibility, however, it was necessary to look at both men and women for a possible common mechanism involving insulin.

1. A Proposed Mechanism

To paraphrase the role of insulin in health, insulin is synthesized in the pancreas and secreted when needed into the blood stream from pancreatic β-cells. During the fed state plasma insulin is elevated, a time when most body cells prefer carbohydrates over other sources of fuel. Insulin allows carbohydrates to enter the cells by attaching first to cell receptors. As the level of plasma insulin subsides, the percentage of fat used for fuel increases while the percentage of carbohydrate used for fuel decreases. Eventually, fats become the preferred fuel type, such as during a fast and during sustained physical exertion. Plasma insulin, during this period, is at its lowest level while the insulin antagonist, glucagon, is at its peak.

Glucagon like insulin, is synthesized in the pancreas, but secreted from pancreatic α-cells rather than from β-cells. The two hormones have a see-saw action. When secretion of one is favored, the other is suppressed. The relative blood level of glucagon and insulin, therefore, serves to dictate at any given moment the preference of the body for fuel, either carbohydrates or fat.

a. The Healthful Process

It is interesting that a high level of plasma glucagon relative to insulin and a high level of HDL, termed "good cholesterol", are both associated with healthful events — the efficient use of fat for fuel, the removal of excess cholesterol from arteries, and a normal TSC. It is equally interesting that HDL particles originate in the liver and in the intestine, the same two sites where glucagon exerts its primary action. This association appears to be more than coincidental, and points to the possibility that factors which elevate plasma glucagon relative to plasma insulin are responsible for initiating the biosynthesis of protective high density lipoprotein (HDL). If research proves this correct it is likely that the amino acid, alanine, is responsible for initiating this process during exercise. Alanine is released from muscle tissue during exercise, the amount of which is directly proportional to the intensity of the work being performed.[19] In fact alanine and glutamine, which are two of the least dominant amino acids in muscle tissue, constitute over 50% of the total amino nitrogen released from exercised muscles. An important purpose is to serve as vehicles for nitrogen and to provide the primary source of blood glucose during exercise. The rise in blood alanine also stimulates release of pancreatic glucagon.[20,21] In this manner alanine plays an important role in integrating the choice of fuel during physical exertion. As the exercise becomes more vigorous, additional alanine is produced which, in turn, stimulates release of additional glucagon. This action sets the stage for the efficient use of fat during this period as the preferred energy substrate. And, as stated before, glucagon appears to be the most important mediator in the biosynthesis of protective HDL.

b. The Atherosclerotic Process

A chronic elevation of fasting plasma insulin and/or an exaggerated insulin response to a glucose load either permits or causes a chronic interference in the normal use of fat for fuel. The excess of insulin relative to glucagon is likely to be a cause for poor mobilization of fats, an unusually low HDL, and the subsequent appearance of an elevated TSC. The extreme of this is identified as insulin resistance and is most often associated with overweight, which likewise associates with a lower HDL, an elevated TSC, and increased heart risk. Furthermore, there is reason to suspect that a chronic excess of insulin relative to glucagon is responsible for the reduction in low density lipoprotein (LDL) receptors that often accompanies an elevated TSC. The work of Thompson helps to explain this scenario;[22] he reported that an inverse relationship exists between low thyroid function and the level of serum insulin. The thyroid activity that accompanies excess insulin inhibits LDL uptake, probably by reducing LDL receptors. These facts make it apparent, therefore, that the task of lowering TSC to reduce heart risk and also to attain optimal health involves more than the simple reduction of diet cholesterol and fat. One must adopt a lifestyle habit of selecting foods that require the least amount of insulin and which stimulate the smallest rise in blood insulin.

c. Diet and Lifestyle

The premise that the smallest insulin excess is an insult to the health of human arteries requires a major adjustment in the manner in which the nutritional value of foods are assessed. Foods cannot be judged simply by their vitamin and caloric content. Foods which are equal in vitamins and calories may differ considerably in the degree to which they effect plasma insulin, body weight, and heart risk. Differences in the insulin response to glucose and fructose, for instance, may explain why fructose is utilized better by both the nondiabetic and diabetic person.[23-25] Crapo, Olefsky, and Jenkins et al.[26-29] have conducted several pilot studies that may lead to a better way for evaluating the influence of a food on both heart health and optimal health. While their works reveal the predictability of the insulin response to a food eaten as a single item, food-combining adds unlimited variables that complicate predictability. Yet, enough work has been done to state with certainty that physical inactivity is the greatest single cause of an elevated fasting insulin. Refined sugar (sucrose) is the second most important factor and the single most important dietary cause of an elevated insulin. Together, a lifestyle of physical inactivity and the habitual consumption of sucrose make a deadly pair. And, in men, when these two factors combine with an excess of estrogen relative to blood testosterone the risk for heart disease may be even greater.

III. HEART DISEASE AND ESTROGEN IN THE MALE

Gerald B. Phillips at Roosevelt Hospital in New York is perhaps the strongest proponent of the theory that, in men, hyperestrogenemia and a reduced testosterone-to-estradiol ratio is the common denominator that links the major risk factors to heart disease.[30-38] Dr. Phillips has noted that while estrogen seems to play a protective role in women, an imbalance in the sex hormone ratio in men is associated with diabetes, being overweight, hypertension, cigarette smoking, and an elevated TSC. "In the Multiple Risk Factor Intervention Trial (MRFIT)," said Phillips, "the levels of blood cholesterol, blood pressure, and cigarette smoking were reduced without any significant reduction in mortality from CHD over seven years." His notation adds support to the premise that one cannot expect to eliminate the cause simply by treating the symptom(s). The exception would be if the symptom and the cause were one and the same. While this is unlikely, the fact remains that an elevated TSC does tend to accelerate the atherosclerotic process and there is much wisdom in trying to lower the TSC. However, much care must be given to the manner in which TSC is lowered. Otherwise, the method employed may not address possible underlying causes. An excellent example is the imbalance in the ratio of male sex hormones that Phillips has noted.

A. A Proposed Mechanism

To paraphrase the role of estrogen in health in the male, 80% of the plasma level of male estrogen is derived from the peripheral metabolism of androgens, occurring mostly in the skin, in the central nervous system, and in adipose tissue. Testosterone is the primary plasma androgen, the concentration of which is about 100 times greater than that of the two primary estrogens, estrone and estradiol. Male sexual behavior is in part dependent upon the stable, 100:1 ratio of testosterone to estrogen. This narrow limit is indirectly under hypothalamus control. Estrogen acts both to inhibit the action of testosterone in particular tissues and in other tissues to enhance its action.

Estrogen in the male is virtually all derived from the catabolism of testosterone. The process seems to be more active with age. Thus, it is normal for the 100:1 ratio of testosterone to estrogen to slowly decline with age. In heart disease, however, there is an increase in the plasma level of estrogen that is greater than the expected change due to aging. Phillips reports that in some of these people feminization can be observed. The consequence is far reaching.

1. The Atherosclerotic Process

Phillips points to the work of Klaiber;[35] he found that an excess of estrogen increases catecholamines, decreases its degradation, and potentiates its action. This combined affect increases the demand of the heart for oxygen, which carries a negative implication for those people with preexisting obstructive coronary artery disease. Cigarette smoking, on the other hand, promotes a higher blood level of the stress hormone, norepinephrine. Plasma norepinephrine may also increase in those people who react poorly to chronic emotional stress. Its adverse action augments the conversion of testosterone to estradiol, thus reducing the ratio. This excess estrogen, Phillips believes, may interfere with the binding of insulin with its receptor, promoting a rise in the fasting level of insulin and promoting an exaggerated insulin response to foods. Conversely, insulin administration may encourage a rise in plasma androgens, which raises the unsettled question of "which came first".

2. Diet and Lifestyle

Overweight can be associated with an elevated plasma insulin. It can also be associated with an excess of estrogen. Insulin, overweight, and estrogen can also be linked with noninsulin-dependent diabetes, which indicates that all four parameters would respond to the same dietary approach. Rosenthal et al.[39] studied the effects of a high-complex-carbohydrate diet in combination with a low fat/low cholesterol diet. The researchers documented a marked reduction in plasma estrogen, TSC, and triglyceride, and a moderate increase in the testosterone-to-estrogen ratio — testoseterone remained the same while estrogen went down. There was also an unfortunate reduction noted for protective HDL, which indicates that while there are measurable benefits from such a diet the optimum diet for correcting this problem still eludes our best intentions.

Regarding cigarette smoking and emotional stress, it is likely that an excess of estrogen prevails over insulin as the underlying factor that associates with heart disease, especially since stress hormones exert an antagonistic effect upon insulin. For these people the solution is quite simple: Stop smoking and learn how best to cope with stress. It is also possible that insulin resistance may develop in other situations secondary to an excess of estrogen. This possibility exists because insulin receptors have been known to be occupied by other hormones. The estrogen excess, therefore, may bind to the receptors of insulin, causing a rise in plasma insulin and a further risk of heart attack.

IV. CHANGING THE FOCUS

While the evidence presented here illustrates that obstructive arterial disease and heart attack may occur without regard to TSC, an elevated TSC remains a very important determinant of heart risk. And the goal of every health practitioner should be to reduce TSC to an acceptable level. The manner in which this is accomplished, however, is very important. The results of the LRC study clearly demonstrate that the low fat/low cholesterol diet as now prescribed may have any one or a combination of five outcomes: it may correct the heart disease problem; it may slow the atherosclerotic process; it may have no effect on preventing a heart attack; it may accomplish nothing other than to redirect the defect to another organ, to manifest as another disease; or it may change the mode of death to an unexpected cause. All of these alternatives may occur in conjunction with a lower TSC, which indicates that the regimen now employed for reducing TSC must be amended before optimum health benefits can be expected. This goal cannot be attained through complacency with our present level of knowledge.

Excesses of insulin and estrogen represent two very important, underlying factors that may cause an elevated TSC. Both may also trigger a rise in serum triglycerides, which likewise has been implicated to some degree in heart disease. An elevated TSC, however, is not an identifying prerequisite of these potential causes of heart disease. Furthermore, an elevated TSC may have reached that level without regard to the quantity of fat and cholesterol in the diet, which questions the wisdom of prescribing an identical lifestyle for everyone. Perhaps there are characteristics about certain sources of fat and cholesterol, or about the way they are gathered and prepared, which become deciding factors that influence either a good outcome or a bad outcome. Many of these possibilities are discussed in this book.

ACKNOWLEDGMENTS

Special thanks to Professor M. F. Oliver, The Duke of Edinburgh Professor of Cardiology, University of Edinburgh (Department of Medicine), Cardiovascular Research Unit, Edinburgh, Scotland, for his review and constructive criticism of the final draft. Also, Gerald B. Phillips, M.D., Roosevelt Hospital, New York, New York, for his review and constructive criticism of the final draft.

REFERENCES

1. The Lipid Research Clinics Coronary Primary Prevention Trial Results. I. Reduction in incidence of coronary heart disease, *JAMA*, 251(3), 351, 1984.
2. Ahrens, E. H., Jr., The diet-heart question in 1985: has it really been settled?, *Lancet*, 1, 1085, 1985.
3. Oliver, M. F., Consensus or nonsensus conferences on coronary heart disease, *Lancet*, 1, 1087, 1985.
4. Beveridge, J. M. R. and Johnson, S. E., Studies on diabetic rats — the production of cardiovascular and renal disease in diabetic rats, *Br. J. Exp. Pathol.*, 31, 285, 1950.
5. Lehner, N. D. M., The effect of insulin deficiency, hypothyroidism, and hypertension on atherosclerosis in the squirrel monkey, *Exp. Mol. Pathol.*, 15, 230, 1971.
6. Kalant, N., Dietary atherogenesis in alloxan diabetes, *J. Lab. Clin. Med.*, 63, 147, 1964.
7. Pierce, F. T., The relationship of serum lipoproteins to atherosclerosis in the cholesterol-fed alloxanized rabbit, *Circulation*, 5, 401, 1952.
8. Kalant, N. and Harland, W. A., The effect of an atherogenic diet on normal and alloxan-diabetic rats, *J. Can. Med. Assoc.*, 84, 251, 1961.
9. Sorge, F., Insulin response to oral glucose in patients with a previous myocardial infarction and in patients with peripheral vascular disease, *Diabetes*, 25(7), 586, 1976.
10. Kashyap, L., Insulin and non-esterified fatty acid metabolism in asymptomatic diabetics and atherosclerotic subjects, *Can. Med. Assoc. J.*, 102, 1165, 1970.
11. Harrison, L. C., Current concepts: insulin resistance in obese diabetic patients, *J. Med. Consult.*, 2, 12, 1979.
12. Stout, R. W., The relationship of abnormal circulating insulin levels to atherosclerosis, *Atherosclerosis*, 27, 1, 1977.
13. Ducimetiere, P., Plasma glucose and insulin levels as coronary heart disease predictors in middle aged active men, in *VIII World Congress of Cardiology*, 1978, 374.
14. Logan, R., Thomson, M., Riemerson, R., and Oliver, M., Risk factors for ischaemic heart-disease in normal men aged 40, *Lancet*, i, 949, 1978.
15. Pyorala, K., Relationship of glucose tolerance and plasma insulin to the incidence of coronary heart disease: results from two population studies in Finland, *Diabetes Care*, 2(2), 131, 1979.
16. Kraft, J., Detection of diabetes mellitus *in situ* (occult diabetes), *Lab. Med.*, 6(2), 10, 1975.
17. Wellborn, T. A. and Wearne, K., Coronary heart disease incidence and mortality in Brusselton with reference to glucose and insulin levels, *Diabetes Care*, 2, 154, 1979.

18. Guerre-Millo, M., Leturgue, A., Girard, J., and Lavau, M., Increased insulin sensitivity and responsiveness of glucose metabolism in adipocytes from female versus male rats, *J. Clin. Invest.*, 76, 109, 1985.
19. Snell, K., Muscle alanine synthesis and hepatic gluconeogenesis, *Biochem. Soc. Trans.*, 8, 205, 1980.
20. Muller, W., Faloona, G., and Unger, R., The effect of alanine on glucagon secretion, *J. Clin. Invest.*, 50, 2215, 1971.
21. Wise, J., Hendler, R., and Felig, P., Evaluation of alpha-cell function by infusion of alanine in normal diabetic and obese subjects, *N. Engl. J. Med.*, 288, 487, 1973.
22. Thompson, G. R., Congenital and acquired defects of receptor-mediated low density lipoprotein catabolism, *Circulation Part II*, 62(4)(Abstr. 146), 44, 1980.
23. Ard, N., Koh, E., Reiser, S., and Knehans, A., Effects of long term feeding of fructose and glucose on lipid parameters, *Fed. Proc. Fed. Am. Soc. Exp. Biol.*, 43, 1063, 1984.
24. Koh, E., and Reiser, S., Effect of long term feeding of fructose and glucose on selected blood parameters, *Fed. Proc. Fed. Am. Soc. Exp. Biol.*, 43, 1064, 1984.
25. Levine, L., Evans, W., Cadarette, B., Fisher, E., and Bullen, B., Fructose and glucose ingestion and muscle glycogen use during submaximal exercise, *J. Appl. Physiol. Respirat. Environ. Exercise Physiol.*, 55(6), 1767, 1983.
26. Crapo, P. and Olefsky, J., Fructose — its characteristics, physiology, and metabolism, *Nutrition Today*, p. 2, July/August, 1980.
27. Crapo, P. and Kolterman, O., The metabolic effects of 2-week fructose feeding in normal subjects, *Am. J. Clin. Nutr.*, 39, 525, 1984.
28. Crapo, P., Scarlett, J., Kolterman, O., Sanders, L., Hofeldt, F., and Olefsky, J., The effects of oral fructose, sucrose, and glucose in subjects with reactive hypoglycemia, *Diabetes Care*, 5(5), 512, 1982.
29. Jenkins, D., Wolever, T., Taylor, R., Barker, H., Harshman, F., Baldwin, J., Bowling, A., Newman, H., Jenkins, A., and Goff, D., Glycemic index of foods: a physiological basis for carbohydrate exchange, *Am. J. Clin. Nutr.*, 34(3), 362, 1981.
30. Phillips, G., Hyperestrogenemia, diet, and disorders of Western Societies, *Am. J. Med.*, 78(3), 363, 1985.
31. Phillips, G., Evidence for hyperestrogenemia as the link between diabetes mellitus and myocardial infarction, *Am. J. Med.*, 76, 1041, 1984.
32. Phillips, G., Sex hormones, risk factors and cardiovascular disease, *Am. J. Med.*, 65, 7, 1978.
33. Phillips, G., Castelli, W., Abbott, R., and McNamara, P., Association of hyperestrogenemia and coronary heart disease in men in the Framingham cohort, *Am. J. Med.*, 74, 863, 1983.
34. Phillips, G., Relationship between serum sex hormones and glucose insulin, and lipid abnormalities in men with myocardial infarction, *Proc. Natl. Acad. Sci.*, 74(4), 1729, 1977.
35. Klaiber, E., Serum estradiol levels in male cigarette smokers, *Am. J. Med.*, 77, 858, 1984.
36. Laskarzewski, P., Morrison, J., Gutal, J., Orchard, T., Khoury, P., and Glueck, C., High and low density lipoprotein cholesterols in adolescent boys: relationships with endogenous testosterone, estradiol, and Quetelet index, *Metabolism*, 32(3), 262, 1983.
37. Schneider, G., Kirschner, M., Berkowitz, R., and Ertel, N., Increased estrogen production in obese men, *J. Clin. Endocrin. Metab.*, 48(4), 633, 1979.
38. Mendoza, S., Zerpa, A., Carrasco, H., Colmenares, O., Rangel, A., Gartside, P., and Kashyap, M., Estradiol, testosterone, apolipoproteins, lipoprotein cholesterol and lipolytic enzymes in men with premature myocardial infarction and angiographically assessed coronary occlusion, *Artery*, 12(1), 1, 1983.
39. Rosenthal, M., Barnard, R., Rose, D., Inkeles, S., Hall, J., and Pritikin, N., Effects of high-complex-carbohydrate, low-fat, low-cholesterol diet on levels of serum lipids and estradiol, *Am. J. Med.*, 78, 23, 1985.

Chapter 3

DIETARY FATS AND THE AGING ADULT

K. K. Willcox and K. Y. Lei

TABLE OF CONTENTS

I. INTRODUCTION

Fats contribute 42% of total kilocalories in the average American diet.[1] This dietary fat is derived largely from animals with roughly three times as much fat coming from animal sources as from vegetable sources.[2] Some foods such as butter, lard, and cooking oils are composed entirely of fat and are referred to as "visible" fats, whereas the less conspicuous forms found in milk, meats, eggs, cereals, and nuts have been termed "hidden" fats.[3] Fats in the diet play several important metabolic roles. Dietary fats contribute palatability to food, and also enhance feelings of satiety since they are slowly digested and delay stomach emptying. As an energy source fats are more concentrated than proteins and carbohydrates and provide approximately 9 kcal/g. Dietary fats also facilitate absorption and transport of the lipid-soluble vitamins A, D, E, and K. Additionally, fats in the diet supply the body with essential fatty acids (EFAs), namely linoleic acid and its relatives, which are necessary for cell membrane integrity and prostaglandin synthesis.[2]

Although fat is an essential nutrient in the diet of humans, consumption of a high level of saturated fat, as is seen in most industrialized nations, has been linked to hypercholesterolemia, accelerated atherosclerosis, and an increased rate of mortality from coronary heart disease (CHD).[4] Numerous risk factors have been identified which are associated with the development of heart disease; these include cigarette smoking, hypertension, and diabetes mellitus.[5] However, of all the major cardiovascular risk factors, only the population mean plasma cholesterol and the intake of both dietary fat and cholesterol are correlated with the incidence and mortality rates from cardiovascular disease.[6] The focus of this chapter will be the consumption of dietary fat by Americans, with particular emphasis on intake by the elderly. The association between dietary fat and cardiovascular disease, as well as age-related changes in dietary fat metabolism, will be addressed.

II. DIETARY FAT INTAKE IN THE U.S.

In the U.S. fat consumption is on the rise. According to data compiled by the U.S. Department of Agriculture (USDA),[7-11] the level of fat in the nation's food supply has increased by more than one third during this century. Data on the Nutrient Content of the U.S. Food Supply indicated that daily per capita consumption of fat rose from 125 g in 1910 to 169 g fat in 1980.[8,9] As a percentage of total kilocalories the contribution of fat has increased from 32% in 1910 to 42% in 1980.[7]

Although the level of fat in the food supply has risen steadily since 1910, the sources of dietary fat have changed considerably during this period. While in 1910 animal fats contributed 83% of total fat kilocalories, in 1980 this amount decreased to 58%. The rise in fat consumption observed between 1910 and 1980 was due primarily to increased use of fats from vegetable sources. Daily per capita consumption of vegetable fats rose from 21.3 g in 1910 to 70.4 g in 1980.[7-9]

Of course it must be noted that figures derived for daily per capita fat consumption represent the total amount of fat available to each individual. Fat waste in food processing, marketing, and home use were only estimated.[7] Perhaps a more accurate estimation of actual fat consumption by individuals can be derived from the USDA Nationwide Food Consumption Survey (NFCS).[10,11] This study reported the amounts and the nutrient content of foods used in entire households as well as by individuals. These figures estimate actual ingestion by individuals rather than the total amount available for ingestion. Consequently, average fat consumption by individuals was reported to be 83 g/day, a level far less than the 169 g derived from the food supply data.[7,10,11]

Data from the NFCS was also analyzed by age groups. In general, fat consumption decreased in males and females between 65 and 74 years as compared to adults in the 35 to 50 year range. However, due to an overall reduction in caloric intake, fat still contributed 41 and 39% of total kilocalories in elderly males and females, repectively. Although these percentages are slightly less than the 43 and 42% reported for middle-aged males and females, respectively,[10,11] the contribution of fat to total caloric intake in the elderly is still above the recommended level proposed by several governmental agencies and professional organizations.[12-16] Analyses of dietary intake in smaller, more selected elderly populations in Vermont[17] and Missouri[18] proved to be in accordance with the data provided by the NFCS.

III. DIGESTION AND ABSORPTION OF FAT IN THE AGING ADULT

Elderly people in the U.S., like their younger counterparts, consume appoximately 40% of their total food energy in the form of fat.[10,11] However, the efficiency of the body in processing dietary fat appears to decline with increasing age. Incomplete fat absorption has been observed in many older people.[19-21] Steatorrhea, or the presence of fat in the stools, was observed in the fecal collections of nearly 40% of 41 adults, ranging in age from 62 to 96 years, who were consuming their normal diet. In these elderly subjects, fat comprised between 20 and 56% of the dried fecal weight, with the majority in the form of undigested triglyceride.[19] Normally, in young adult subjects fecal fat comprises less than 10% of dried fecal weight and when found is predominantly in fatty acid form.[22]

The amount of fat fed at one meal influences the degree of both digestion and absorption of the nutrient. Swedes ranging in age from 67 to 72 years were given an oral fat load of 115 g. Fecal fat was found largely in the form of triglyceride and ranged from 5 to 16 g for the elderly as compared to 3 to 9 g for young controls.[21] When the same amount of fat (115 g) was distributed across all meals and snacks, fecal fat in the elderly dropped to 5 to 7 g and was equal to that found in young controls.[21]

Nutrient absorption is dependent on many factors, among them pancreatic enzyme secretion, blood supply to the absorption site, and integrity of the intestinal mucosa.[23] Although a reduction in mucosal surface area has been observed in aging humans,[24] its effects on absorption and transport capacity have not been clearly identified.[25] Several studies examining fat digestion in the elderly have indicated that impaired fat absorption can be largely attributed to a reduction in pancreatic lipase secretion.[20,26] Pancreatic lipase is necessary for the hydrolysis of fats into fatty acids and monoacylglycerides, forms which are readily absorbed by the mucosal surface of the small intestine.[2] The presence of triglyceride fats, rather than fatty acids, in the stools of older adults suggests that malabsorption may be due to an inability to hydrolyse fats so that absorption is not facilitated. This hypothesis is supported by data from a study involving 43 elderly men ranging in age from 66 to 96 years. After a 100 g oral fat load, a peak in plasma lipids occurred approximately 5 hr later in the elderly subjects as compared to 3 hr for young control subjects. When a pancreatic extract was administered with the fat load, the peak in blood lipid levels occurred at similar times in both young and old subjects.[20] Thus, the malabsorption observed in elderly subjects may have resulted largely from a pancreatic insufficiency in the production of lipase.

IV. DIETARY FAT AND CORONARY HEART DISEASE (CHD)

Diseases of the vascular system, particularly cardiovascular disease, currently account for over 50% of all deaths in the U.S. each year.[27] This trend is not restricted to the U.S. however, since a large proportion of the mortality and morbidity in most industrialized nations has been attributed to cardiovascular disease.[2] Much has been written about the role which nutrition might play as a factor in causing vascular disease or at least in influencing its progression. Dietary fat intake is one nutritional factor that has been associated with elevated plasma cholesterol and accelerated atherosclerosis and CHD.[28] This association has been based on a wide variety of epidemiological, clinical and experimental studies.

The World Health Organization (WHO) and Food and Agricultural Organization (FAO) have provided statistics from 30 countries that indicate a positive correlation between mortality and intake of total kilocalories, total fat, animal fat, meat, cholesterol, eggs, and animal protein in men 55 to 59 years of age; there is either no correlation or a negative correlation between CHD and intake of vegetable fat, vegetables, and fish.[29] A positive association between dietary saturated fat intake and atherosclerotic disease has also been shown in other epidemiologic studies. The International Co-operative Study on Epidemiology of Cardiovascular Disease, a prospective study of 40- to 59-year-old men from seven countries, revealed that the percentage of total calories provided by saturated fat correlates significantly with the incidence of myocardial infarction. Additionally, a direct relationship existed between serum cholesterol levels and consumption of saturated fat as well as the incidence of myocardial infarction.[30]

Changes in dietary habits, particularly in the increased consumption of saturated animal fats and cholesterol, can also result in an increased incidence of coronary artery disease. Gordon[31,32] first described a gradient in mortality from heart disease in Japanese men living in Japan, Hawaii, and California. Of all the industrialized countries in the world, Japan has one of the lowest rates of CHD, less than 150 deaths per 100,000 males aged 55 to 59.[29] However, this value increases as Japanese men are assimilated into the westernized society of the U.S. Deaths resulting from CHD increased threefold in men living in California as compared to their counterparts in Japan. A comparison of food consumption between the populations revealed that a number of dietary parameters followed a similar pattern. In particular, intake of total protein, total fat, and cholesterol were highest in the California population and lowest in the Japanese population.[33]

In addition to human epidemiological studies, animal experimentation has revealed a relationship between fat intake, plasma cholesterol levels, and both the development and severity of atherosclerosis.[34] Research on this topic was first reported in 1913 when it was found that a saturated fat-rich diet induced atherosclerosis in rabbits.[35] Since then it has been shown that full-blown atherosclerosis leading to myocardial infarction can be induced in nearly every type of laboratory animal simply by feeding a diet which elevates plasma cholesterol levels.[36-39]

The type of fat ingested appears to be equally if not more important than the quantity of fat consumed as far as hyperlipidemia, atherosclerosis, and heart disease is concerned. Prior to 1950, the total fat content of the diet was considered to be the controlling factor in determining plasma cholesterol levels and an individual's risk of developing heart disease. However, in the early 1950s a differential effect of saturated and polyunsaturated fats on plasma cholesterol levels was discovered. In that year Kinsell[40] reported that animal fats increased the plasma cholesterol level while vegetable fats lowered it. A positive correlation between the degree of dietary fat unsaturation and its ability to lower plasma cholesterol was also observed.[41] Gram for gram, saturated fats were about twice as effective in raising the plasma cholesterol level in man as polyunsaturated fats were in lowering it, with monounsaturated fats neutral in their effect.[41] Similar responses to the degree of dietary fat saturation have been observed in animal models.[42]

The opposing effects of polyunsaturated and saturated fats on plasma cholesterol levels have led to the proposal of possible mechanisms responsible for the observed differences. In 1970, Grundy and Ahrens[43] listed four possible mechanisms responsible for the hypocholesterolemic effects of dietary polyunsaturated fat: decreased intestinal absorption of cholesterol, decreased synthesis of endogenous cholesterol, an increased excretion of fecal neutral and acidic steroids, and a redistribution of cholesterol from plasma to tissues. More recent work has suggested that rates of lipoprotein synthesis and/or catabolism are changed when polyunsaturated fat is fed, and that the degree of saturation of the ingested triglyceride affects the cholesterol-carrying capacity of lipoproteins.[44,45] A more detailed review of the effects of polyunsaturated fats on cholesterol metabolism is presented in another chapter.

Finally, apart from epidemiological studies and animal experiments, several large-scale, long-term nutritional intervention trials have been performed to study the possible beneficial effects of dietary manipulation.[46-50] Most of these studies involved substitution of a large percentage of animal fat with polyunsaturated fat and one of these studies also involved drastic reductions in cholesterol intake.[47] Nutritional modification appears to provide little or no improvement except for a reduction in cardiovascular events and total mortality for a subgroup of men under 50 years of age in one of the studies.[47] However, this reduction disappeared when men of all ages were compared. Thus the data from these human studies do not sanction the drastic alteration of the typical American diet, especially for the elderly population. Although nutritional intervention may not provide appreciable benefits late in life, Hazzard in a review of aging and atherosclerosis emphasized that intervention should be initiated early in life and implemented on a life-long basis.[51]

V. SUMMARY

The consumption of saturated fats is associated with an increased risk for developing cardiovascular disease. This association is based largely on epidemiological surveys which compared lifestyle trends, in particular dietary patterns, with the rate of mortality from CHD.[52] The evidence obtained from these studies in no way conclusively demonstrates a causative relationship between dietary fat and heart disease.[53] Rather, an indirect relationship exists whereby diets rich in saturated fat tend to increase total plasma cholesterol levels in some individuals, which in itself is a major risk factor for the development of atherosclerosis.[34] However, fat content of the diet is only one factor which influences plasma cholesterol levels. Total calories, protein and carbohydrate content, and dietary fiber intake are other nutritional factors which can influence plasma cholesterol levels. Therefore, caution must be exercised before encouraging widespread use of a low fat, low cholesterol diet in order to combat cardiovascular disease.[54]

In 1977, the U.S. Senate Select Committee on Nutrition and Human Needs issued a report that outlined specific guidelines for Americans which would aid in the prevention of CHD.[12] One recommendation called for a reduction in the amount of saturated fat and cholesterol consumed by Americans. This report helped to establish a public health policy on the role of fats in the development of CHD. This policy, known as the diet-heart hypothesis, has not met with uniform approval since conclusive evidence for a causative relationship between dietary fat intake and heart disease has not yet been established.[53] While low fat diets may result in lower plasma cholesterol levels in some individuals, it is unwise to prescribe dietary modifications for entire population groups. Rather, individuals at a higher risk for coronary heart disease, for example people with cholesterol levels exceeding 250 mg/dℓ, could be identified and advised to reduce the consumption of fat in an effort to reduce plasma cholesterol.[52] However, other investigators contend that the type of fat consumed, rather than the amount, is the important factor in determining whether or not cardiovascular disease will develop. Instead of encouraging the use of a low fat diet, Sinclair[55] stresses the importance of maintaining a high ratio of essential (polyunsaturated) to nonessential fatty acids in the diet to reduce total plasma cholesterol levels. Other investigators emphasize that risk factors such as cigarette smoking and hypertension must also be evaluated, along with dietary patterns, to determine the degree to which they promote the development of heart disease.[56]

Conflicting opinions on the role of fats in cardiovascular disease make the diet-heart hypothesis a controversial issue. Scientists and clinicians alike question the advisability of prescribing a low-saturated fat diet to the general public for the purpose of reducing cardiovascular disease, especially when the long-term effects of this dietary modification have not yet been established.[52] The public should be made aware of the controversy surrounding this issue so that individuals can make informed choices regarding their diet and how it applies to their health.

REFERENCES

1. U.S. Senate Committee on Nutrition and Human Needs, *Dietary Goals for the United States,* U.S. Government Printing Office, 1977.
2. Gurr, M. I., in *Role of Fats in Food and Nutrition,* Elsevier, Amsterdam, 1984, 61.
3. Robson, J. R. K., Larkin, F. A., Sandretto, A. M., and Tadayon, B., *Malnutrition Causation and Control,* Gordon Breach Science Publications, 1972.
4. Wissler, R. W. and McGill, H. C., Conference on blood lipids in children: optimal levels for early prevention of coronary artery disease, *Prev. Med.,* 12, 868, 1983.
5. Havel, R. J., Goldstein, J. L., and Brown, M. S., Lipoprotein and lipid transport, in *Metabolic Control and Disease,* 8th ed., Bondy, P. K. and Rosenberg, L. E., Eds., W. B. Saunders, Philadelphia, 1980, 393.
6. Keys, A., *Seven Countries: A Multivariate Analysis of Death and Coronary Heart Disease,* Harvard University Press, Cambridge, 1980.
7. Rizek, R. L., Welsh, S. O., Marsten, R. M., and Jackson, E. M., Levels and sources of fat in the U.S. food supply and in diets of individuals, in *Dietary Fats and Health,* Perkins, E. G. and Visek, W. J., Eds., Amercian Oil Chemists' Soceity, Champaign, Illinois, 1981, 13.
8. USDA Consumer and Food Economics Research Division, Food Consumption, Prices and Expenditures, Economics Research Service, Agric. Econ. Rep No. 138, U.S. Department of Agriculture, Washington, D.C.
9. USDA Consumer Nutrition Center, Food Consumption, Prices and Expenditures, Economics and Statistics Service, Statistical Bulletin No. 656, U.S. Department of Agriculture, Washington, D.C., 1981.
10. USDA, Science and Education Administration, Consumer Nutrition Center, Nutrient Levels in Food Used by Households in the United States, Nationwide Food Consumption Survey, 1977-78, Preliminary Report No. 3, U.S. Department of Agriculture, Washington, D.C., 1981.
11. USDA, Science and Education Administration, Consumer Nutrition Center, Food and Nutrient Intakes of Individuals in One Day in the United States, Nationwide Food Consumption Survey, 1977-1978, Preliminary Report No. 2, U.S. Department of Agriculture, Washington, D.C., 1980.
12. Select Committee on Nutrition and Human Needs, *U.S. Senate Dietary Goals for the United States,* 2nd ed., U.S. Government Printing Office, Washington, D.C., No. 052-070-04376-8, 1977.
13. USDA-DHEW, Nutrition and Your Health-Dietary Guidelines for Americans, U.S. Department of Agriculture and Department of Health, Education, and Welfare, Washington, D.C., 1980.
14. U.S. Department of Health, Education, and Welfare, *Healthy People: The Surgeon General's Report on Health Promotion and Disease Prevention,* U.S. Government Printing Office, Washington, D.C., No. 79-55071, 1979.
15. NAS, National Research Council, Food and Nutritional Board, Toward Healthful Diets, National Academy of Sciences, Washington, D.C., 1980.

16. American Medical Association, Council on scientific affairs, concept of nutrition and health, *JAMA*, 242, 2335, 1979.
17. Clarke, R. R., Schlenker, E. D., and Merrow, S. B., Nutrient intake, adiposity, plasma total cholesterol, and blood pressure of rural participants in the (Vermont) Nutrition Program for Older Americans (Title III), *Am. J. Clin. Nutr.*, 34, 1743, 1981.
18. Kohrs, M. B., O'Neal, R., Preston, A., Eklund, D., and Abrahams, O., Nutritional status of elderly residents in Missouri, *Am. J. Clin. Nutr.*, 31, 2186, 1978.
19. Pelz, K. S., Gottfried, S. P., and Soos, E., Intestinal absorption studies in the aged, *Geriatrics*, 23, 149, 1968.
20. Webster, S. G., Wilkinson, E. M., and Gowland, E., A comparison of fat absorption in young and old subjects, *Age Aging*, 6, 113, 1977.
21. Werner, I. and Hambraeus, L., The digestive capacity of elderly people, in *Nutrition in Old Age*, Carlson, L. A., Ed., Symposia Swedish Nutrition Foundation X, Almquist & Wiksell, Stockholm.
22. Schlenker, E. D., Nutrient digestion and absorption, in *Nutrition and Aging*, C. V. Mosby, St. Louis, 1984.
23. Geokas, M. C. and Haverback, B. J., The aging gastrointestinal tract, *Am. J. Surg.*, 117, 881, 1969.
24. Warren, P. M., Pepperman, M. A., and Montgomery, R. D., Age changes in small-intestinal mucosa, *Lancet*, 2, 849, 1978.
25. Holt, P. R., Effects of aging upon intestinal absorption, in *Nutritional Approaches to Aging Research*, Moment, G. B., Ed., CRC Press, Boca Raton, Fla., 1982, 127.
26. Becker, G. H., Meyer, J., and Necheles, H., Fat absorption in young and old age, *Gastroenterology*, 14, 80, 1950.
27. Mahley, R. W., Cellular and molecular biology of lipoprotein metabolism in atherosclerosis, *Diabetes*, 30, 60, 1981.
28. Mahley, R. W., The role of dietary fat and cholesterol in atherosclerosis and lipoprotein metabolism, *West J. Med.*, 134, 34, 1981.
29. Connor, W. E. and Connor, S. L., The key role of nutritional factors in the prevention of coronary heart disease, *Prev. Med.*, 1, 49, 1972.
30. Keys, A., Coronary heart disease — the global picture, *Atherosclerosis*, 22, 149, 1975.
31. Gordon, T., Mortality experience among the Japanese in the United States, Hawaii and Japan, *Public Health Rep.*, 72, 543, 1957.
32. Gordon, T., Further mortality experience among Japanese Americans, *Public Health Rep.*, 82, 973, 1967.
33. Tillotson, J. L., Kato, H., Nichaman, M. Z., Epidemiology of coronary heart disease and stroke in Japanese men living in Japan, Hawaii and California: methodology for comparison of diet, *Am. J. Clin. Nutr.*, 26, 177, 1973.
34. Glueck, C. J., Dietary fat and atherosclerosis, *Am. J. Clin. Nutr.*, 32, 2703, 1979.
35. Anitschkow, N. and Chalatow, S., On experimental cholesterin steatosis and its significance in the origin of some pathological processes, *Arteriosclerosis*, 3, 178, 1983.
36. Wissler, R. W., Development of the atherosclerotic plaque, in *The Myocardium: Failure and Infarction*, Braunwald, E., Ed., H. P. Publishing, New York, 1973, 155.
37. Blaton, V. and Peeters, H., The nonhuman primates as models for studying human atherosclerosis: studies on the chimpanzee, the baboon and the rhesus macacus, in *Atherosclerosis Drug Discovery*, Day, C. E., Ed., Plenum Press, New York, 1976, 33.
38. Ross, R. and Harker, L., Hyperlipidemia and atherosclerosis, *Science*, 193, 1094, 1976.
39. Stills, H. F., and Clarkson, T. B., Atherosclerosis, in *Spontaneous Animal Models of Human Disease*, Andrews, E. J., et al., Eds., Vol. 1, Academic Press, New York, 1979, 70.
40. Kinsel, L. W., Partridge, J., Boling, L., Margen, S., and Michaels, G. P., Dietary modification of serum cholesterol and phospholipid levels, *J. Clin. Endocrinol.*, 12, 909, 1952.
41. Keys, A., Anderson, J. T., and Grande, F., Prediction of serum-cholesterol responses of man to changes in fats in the diet, *Lancet*, 2, 959, 1957.
42. Mahley, R. W., Dietary fat, cholesterol and accelerated atherosclerosis, *Atheroscler. Rev.*, 5, 1, 1979.
43. Grundy, S. M. and Ahrens, E. H., Jr., The effects of unsaturated dietary fats on absorption, excretion, synthesis and distribution of cholesterol in man, *J. Clin. Invest.*, 49, 1135, 1970.
44. Hopkins, P. N. and Williams, R. R., A simplified approach to lipoprotein kinetics and factors affecting serum cholesterol and triglyceride concentrations, *Am. J. Clin. Nutr.*, 34, 2560, 1981.
45. Goodnight, S. H., Jr., Harris, W. S., Connor, W. E., and Illingworth, D. R., Polyunsaturated fatty acids, hyperlipidemia, and thrombosis, *Arteriosclerosis*, 2, 87, 1982.
46. National Diet-Heart Study, Final report, *Circulation*, 37(Suppl. 1), 1, 1968.
47. Brewer, E. R., Ashman, P. L., and Kuba, K., Minnesota Coronary Survey — composition of diets, adherence and serum-lipid response, *Circulation*, 52, 269, 1975.

48. Frantz, I. D., Jr., Dawson, E. A., Kuba, K., Brewer, E. R., Gatewood, L. C., and Bartsch, G. E., Minnesota Coronary Survey — effect of diet on cardiovascular events and deaths, *Circulation,* 52, 4, 1975.
49. Miettinen, M., Effect of cholesterol-lowering diet on mortality from coronary heart disease and other causes. A 12-year clinical trial in men and women, *Lancet,* 2, 835, 1972.
50. Dayton, S., Chapman, J. M., Pearce, M. L., and Popjak, G. J., Cholesterol, atherosclerosis, ischemic heart disease, and stroke, *Ann. Intern. Med.,* 72, 97, 1970.
51. Hazzard, W. R., Aging and atherosclerosis: interactions with diet, heredity and associated risk factors, in *Nutrition, Longevity, and Aging,* Rockstein, M. and Sussman, M. L., Eds., Academic Press, New York, 1977, 143.
52. Glueck, C. J., Appraisal of dietary fat as a causative factor in atherogenesis, *Am. J. Clin. Nutr.,* 32, 2637, 1979.
53. Hulley, S. B., Sherwin, R., Nestle, M., and Lee, P. R., Epidemiology as a guide to clinical decisions. II. Diet and coronary heart disease: another view. *West. J. Med.,* 135, 25, 1981.
54. Glueck, C. J., Mattson, F. and Bierman, E. L., Diet and coronary heart disease: another view, *N. Eng. J. Med.,* 298, 1471, 1978.
55. Sinclair, H., Dietary fats and coronary heart disease, *Lancet,* 1, 414, 1980.
56. Dwyer, T. and Hetzel, B. S., A comparison of trends of coronary heart disease mortality in Australia, USA and England and Wales with reference to three major risk factors — hypertension, cigarette smoking and diet, *Int. J. Epidemiol.,* 9, 65, 1980.

Chapter 4

NUTRITION AND CHOLESTEROL METABOLISM

Donald J. McNamara

TABLE OF CONTENTS

I. INTRODUCTION

It has been known for over 25 years that a number of dietary factors can significantly influence plasma lipoprotein cholesterol concentrations. Dietary recommendations to the public have become a cornerstone of the mass intervention approach to lower plasma cholesterol levels and, in theory, to reduce the incidence of cardiovascular disease. Studies investigating the mechanisms by which dietary constituents affect plasma cholesterol levels have been directed toward the measurement of their effect on plasma lipoprotein metabolism and on the key parameters of cholesterol homeostasis in the body — intake and absorption, synthesis and catabolism, fecal excretion, and tissue flux.

The sterol balance method, originally developed by Ahrens and co-workers at the Rockefeller University,[1-5] has been the predominant technique used to measure whole body cholesterol metabolism in man. Application of this technique, under controlled metabolic ward conditions, has provided most of the data defining the interaction of dietary factors and endogenous cholesterol metabolism in man. Analysis of plasma cholesterol isotope kinetics, either by compartmental analysis[6] or input-output analysis,[7] has enabled clinical investigators to determine the effects of plasma cholesterol lowering dietary interventions on cholesterol turnover (i.e, the sum of endogenous synthesis and absorbed dietary cholesterol) and pool sizes and, when combined with sterol balance techniques,[8] to fully characterize the key parameters of whole body cholesterol homeostasis in a patient prior to and following institution of a specific dietary intervention.

II. CHOLESTEROL METABOLISM

A. General Aspects

Whole body cholesterol metabolism is a complex interplay of a number of metabolic processes: dietary cholesterol intake and absorption; biliary cholesterol output and reabsorption; endogenous cholesterol synthesis in the liver and other body tissues; cholesterol catabolism to bile acids, the major catabolic endproduct; fecal excretion of cholesterol, bile acids, and their secondary bacterial products; and the influx and efflux of cholesterol between the plasma compartment and the tissues of the body.

An average 70-kg man has a total body cholesterol pool of 145 g; 45 g in the central nervous system, which is relatively inert in terms of whole body metabolism, and 100 g distributed throughout the body tissues and plasma. At any time approximately 5.5% of the body's total pool of cholesterol exists in the plasma compartment. Assuming a daily intake of 440 mg of dietary cholesterol and a 50% absorption, this average man obtains 220 mg/day of cholesterol from his diet. At the same time he is synthesizing 11 mg/kg/day (770 mg) for a total input (turnover) from dietary sources and endogenous production of 990 mg/day. The body's metabolic requirements for cholesterol will utilize about 250 mg/day for bile acid production and steroid hormones, which leaves our average man with the burden of disposing of a cholesterol excess of 740 mg/day. This excess is disposed of by fecal excretion of unabsorbed biliary cholesterol and bile acids (Table 1).

With a balance of cholesterol inputs (absorbed exogenous dietary and endogenous synthesis) and outputs (catabolism and fecal excretion), plasma cholesterol levels remain relatively constant; however, any alteration in this balance can result in either an increase in plasma cholesterol levels or, more importantly, a change in the flux of cholesterol between tissue pools. Those factors causing an increased efflux or a decreased influx of tissue cholesterol would be considered beneficial; in contrast, any

Table 1
CHOLESTEROL MASS AND
METABOLISM IN MAN

Total body cholesterol pool	145 g
Metabolically active pool	100 g
Plasma cholesterol pool	6.5 g
Dietary cholesterol intake	0.5 g/day
Absorbed dietary cholesterol	0.22 g/day
Endogenous cholesterol synthesis	0.77 g/day
Absorbed plus synthesized	0.99 g/day
Metabolic requirement	0.25 g/day
Excess	0.74 g/day

Note: Calculated for a 70-kg man with a plasma cholesterol of 210 mg/dℓ.

intervention resulting in an increased influx or decreased efflux of cholesterol may be harmful. As will be seen later, significant changes in the flux of cholesterol between tissues can occur in the absence of quantitative changes in plasma cholesterol levels. Thus it cannot be assumed that the absence of change in plasma levels negates potential changes in tissue cholesterol stores. As described below, some individuals have exceptionally precise regulatory mechanisms which allow their metabolism to compensate for alterations in this overall balance of cholesterol inputs and outputs and results in stable plasma levels and tissue stores of cholesterol. On the other hand, there are those patients who fail to effectively compensate for perturbations of the system, the result being increased plasma cholesterol levels and/or increased accumulation of cholesterol in body tissues.

It is important to determine not only what effects a dietary constituent may have on plasma cholesterol levels but also what effects a specific dietary constituent may have on whole body cholesterol metabolism and pool sizes. More importantly, by analysis of sterol balance it is possible to determine in which patients the intervention will be effective since the heterogeneity of metabolic reponses in man, which is well established, precludes generalizations in terms of a specific patient's response to dietary change. Sterol balance and pool size data enable the clinical investigator to understand not only the pattern of the plasma lipid changes but also the mechanism of action and potential benefit that might accrue from addition or deletion of a specific dietary factor.

B. Techniques

Whole body cholesterol metabolism in humans is most accurately determined by sterol balance methods, either isotopic, chromatographic, or a combination of the two.[5] The sterol balance method is based on the premise that the sum of fecal neutral (i.e., cholesterol) and acidic (i.e., bile acids) steroid excretion, minus dietary cholesterol intake, equals endogenous cholesterol synthesis. This definition is true only during the metabolic steady state, as described below. Combination of the original balance technique with analysis of plasma cholesterol kinetics makes possible the measurement of endogenous cholesterol synthesis (balance) and turnover (sum of absorbed dietary and endogenous synthesis of cholesterol) and the total exchangeable, metabolically active mass of cholesterol in the body.[8] A combination of these two techniques provides a complete characterization of the effects of a specific dietary factor on cholesterol metabolism and pool size and enables investigators to better define the role of diet in determining plasma cholesterol levels and whole body cholesterol metabolism.

C. Metabolic Studies

Any attempt to measure whole body cholesterol balance in man is complicated by two variables: bacterial breakdown of cholesterol to a variety of neutral steroids in the intestinal tract, and variations in fecal flow rates. Two correction factors are employed to account for these variables: recovery of the nonabsorbable plant sterol sitosterol, which is metabolized and degraded by the intestinal bacteria at a rate identical to cholesterol,[3] and recovery of the fecal flow marker chromic oxide, which is given daily during the balance measurement for determining daily fecal output.[4] In order for these markers to be quantitative it is necessary to establish a constant intake and fecal output of both standards prior to carrying out the actual sterol balance measurements.

In addition to the two fecal markers, a primary criteria for accurate sterol balance measurements of cholesterol synthesis is that the patient be in a "metabolic steady state", i.e., that there is no flux of cholesterol into or out of body tissues. The "metabolic steady state" requirement for sterol balance studies is difficult to validate since it cannot be measured directly. As an arbitrary definition, a "steady state" is assumed to exist when the patient's weight, plasma lipid levels, and fecal output of neutral and acidic steroids remain constant during the period of sterol balance measurement. Even with satisfaction of these arbitrary criteria it is conceivable that a given intervention may appear to maintain a "steady state" while in fact dramatically altering tissue cholesterol flux. Under such conditions the balance measurements either underestimate cholesterol synthesis due to influx or overestimate the true rate due to efflux of tissue cholesterol and its excretion in the feces.

Since most diets contain some cholesterol it is necessary to determine both endogenous synthesis of cholesterol and dietary cholesterol intake and absorption in order to fully characterize the metabolic response to a specific dietary factor. Measurement of cholesterol absorption can be performed by a variety of methods,[9-15] both isotopic and nonisotopic. These techniques require either collection and analysis of fecal samples, nasogastric intubation, and/or intravenous infusion of radiolabeled cholesterol tracers. Most of these techniques provide information on the percent absorption of dietary cholesterol and not the actual amount of cholesterol absorbed. Cholesterol absorption varies significantly between individuals with an average absorption of 55% and a range of 20 to 85%,[16] yet is relatively constant within the same patient.[11,14] Studies have shown that most patients have higher rates of absorption of endogenous biliary cholesterol than of exogenous dietary cholesterol.[15] Most techniques for measuring cholesterol absorption specifically quantitate absorption of exogenous dietary cholesterol.

Cholesterol synthesis can be calculated from the difference between fecal neutral and acidic sterol output and dietary cholesterol intake, irrespective of the fractional absorption of dietary cholesterol (chromatographic balance). Measurement of cholesterol turnover requires analysis of dietary cholesterol intake and absorption, and the rate of cholesterol synthesis (combined isotopic and chromatographic balance).[5] Measurement of cholesterol turnover provides data on the total input of cholesterol (absorbed plus synthesized) and is an important characterization of the total metabolic response of a patient to a dietary or drug intervention.

D. Generalizations

There are some generalized findings regarding whole body cholesterol metabolism in man:

- The average rate of whole body cholesterol synthesis in men and women of normal body weight and normal triglyceride levels is 11 mg/kg/day irrespective of plasma cholesterol levels.

- The average absorption of dietary cholesterol is 55%.
- Hypertriglyceridemic patients have elevated rates of whole body cholesterol synthesis.
- Obese patients have elevated rates of whole body cholesterol synthesis.
- The rate of bile acid synthesis averages 3.5 mg/kg/day in normolipidemic patients.
- The rate of sterol loss via the skin averages 1.2 mg/kg/day, of which 0.4 mg is derived from plasma cholesterol.[17]
- The cholesterol concentration in connective tissues (but not in muscle, adipose or skin) increases with age.[18]

III. DIETARY EFFECTS ON CHOLESTEROL METABOLISM

A. Total Calories

Obesity is associated with an over-production of cholesterol which can be reduced to within the normal range by weight reduction.[19-22] This characteristic of the obese patient is independent of his or her plasma lipid and lipoprotein levels and does not depend on the presence of hyperlipidemia. Each kilogram of excess body weight results in an increase in the rate of cholesterol synthesis of 22 mg/day.[23] This increased production of cholesterol in obesity is accompanied by an increased secretion of cholesterol in the bile leading to supersaturation of bile and increased risk of gallstone formation.[24] Plasma cholesterol isotope kinetic studies of whole body cholesterol metabolism in a large population of patients with various body weights, percent ideal body weights, and plasma lipid levels, have shown that the major determinant of the cholesterol production rate is body weight, and that body weight is directly related to the mass of the total exchangeable pool of cholesterol in the body.[25]

B. Dietary Fats
1. Cholesterol

To many people, the cholesterol in their diet and the cholesterol in their blood are directly related, and dietary cholesterol is the primary source of plasma cholesterol. The fact is that the body's production of cholesterol greatly exceeds the amount of cholesterol most individuals absorb from their diet; exogenous dietary cholesterol accounts for only 20% of the total daily cholesterol input, with the remaining 80% coming from endogenous synthesis. Humans, like a number of animal species, have the ability to feedback regulate endogenous cholesterol synthesis when the intake of dietary cholesterol is increased. Most studies attempting to study the effect of dietary cholesterol on whole body cholesterol metabolism have increased dietary cholesterol intake to such a large extent that it is generally assumed that high cholesterol diets increase plasma cholesterol levels. When dietary cholesterol intake is increased from very low levels to 1 to 3.5 g/day, the absorbed dietary cholesterol input increases to 550 to 2000 mg/day, which can exceed the basal endogenous synthesis rate; thus, the increased cholesterol intake completely overwhelms the synthetic capacity and probably the feedback compensatory ability of the system.

One of the first demonstrations that regulation of endogenous cholesterol synthesis occurs in man was the report that blockage of cholesterol absorption by oral administration of the plant sterol sitosterol, resulted in a significant increase in the rate of whole body cholesterol synthesis.[26] Subsequent studies demonstrated that the two primary metabolic responses to an increase in absorbed dietary cholesterol were (1) increased biliary and fecal re-excretion of absorbed dietary cholesterol, and (2) a feedback suppression of endogenous sterol synthesis.[27] This study also illustrated the extent of metabolic heterogeneity in regulatory responses in man; some patients were effective re-excretors, some effective feedback regulators, some were both, and some were neither.[27] The results clearly showed that some patients could effectively compensate for a large increase in dietary cholesterol while others were noncompensators, unable to handle a cholesterol challenge. This report also provided the first evidence that net tissue accumulation of cholesterol does occur in some patients on a high cholesterol diet, even in the absence of an increase in plasma cholesterol levels.

A high dietary cholesterol intake (3.1 to 3.4 g/day) has been shown to increase hepatic cholesterol concentrations (256 mg/g w/w in controls vs. 417 mg/g w/w in cholesterol-fed patients), indicative of net tissue influx of cholesterol.[28] These studies investigated not only the metabolic response to a high cholesterol diet but also the metabolic responses once the high cholesterol intake had been stopped.[28] The results demonstrated that following cessation of a cholesterol-rich diet, a variety of metabolic responses occurred in individual patients: (1) increased fecal bile acid output, suggesting that one response is an increased catabolism to and excretion of fecal acidic sterols; (2) increased fecal neutral steroid excretion, indicative of efflux of accumulated tissue stores; (3) reduced fecal steroid excretion upon shifting to a lower cholesterol diet, suggestive of a persistence of feedback suppression from the original dietary cholesterol challenge; and (4) no change in total sterol balance as compared to the initial control values. The extent of these various responses, and their precision, were unrelated to the patient's plasma cholesterol level during the initial and final control periods or during intake of the high cholesterol diets.

In a similar series of investigations, Maranhao and Quintao[29] studied a group of patients with a range of plasma cholesterol levels to determine if the metabolic responses to an increase in dietary cholesterol (1350 mg/day) were related to the patient's type of hypercholesterolemia. Their results showed that the ability, or inability, to compensate for a dietary cholesterol challenge is not related to the individual's plasma cholesterol level. As found in previous studies, the results demonstrated that patients responded to the cholesterol challenge in a variety of ways: increased re-excretion of absorbed cholesterol, increased fecal bile acid excretion, decreased endogenous cholesterol synthesis, net tissue accumulation, and combinations of all four compensatory responses. The most consistent finding of this study was that the majority of patients who exhibited no increase in plasma cholesterol levels upon intake of the high cholesterol diet had significant reductions in endogenous sterol synthesis rates. The results are similar to findings of Nestel and Poyser[30] and support the concept that patients with the most effective feedback suppression of cholesterol synthesis are relatively resistant to increases in plasma cholesterol levels.

Studies feeding more modest amounts of cholesterol have been reported by Nestel and Poyser[30] who further confirmed the existence of precise feedback control mechanisms in man. Increasing dietary cholesterol intake from 250 to 750 mg/day resulted in an increase in absorbed dietary cholesterol of 230 mg/day and compensatory responses (increased re-excretion and decreased synthesis of cholesterol) equal to 226 mg/day. Thus, the increment in absorbed dietary cholesterol was completely balanced by the body's regulatory mechanisms. Interestingly, an apparent precision in overall compensatory responses did not prevent an increase in plasma cholesterol levels; cholesterol levels increased the most in one third of the subjects who expressed the smallest suppression of endogenous cholesterol synthesis even though these patients had significant re-excretion of adsorbed dietary cholesterol. The authors hypothesize that increased biliary re-excretion of absorbed dietary cholesterol occurs when feedback suppression of endogenous synthesis fails to effectively function as a compensatory mechanism causing an increase in plasma cholesterol levels.

Studies of the effect of dietary cholesterol intake on sterol metabolism in freshly isolated human blood mononuclear leukocytes[31,32] add further support to the evidence for feedback suppression of cholesterol synthesis in man. When patients are fed low and then high cholesterol diets, both acetate incorporation into sterols and the specific activity of the rate limiting enzyme of sterol synthesis, 3-hydroxy-3-methylglutaryl-CoA reductase, are significantly reduced in mononuclear leukocytes. These results suggest that dietary cholesterol suppresses endogenous cholesterol synthesis in most cholesterol-producing tissues including the peripheral cells of the body.

Studies of the feedback regulation of cholesterol synthesis in a population habituated to a low cholesterol diet have been reported by McMurry et al.[33] The Tarahumara Indians of Mexico have a basal sterol metabolism which is significantly different from that of the average American; lower percent absorption of cholesterol and a higher total cholesterol turnover due to an increased bile acid synthesis rate. When study subjects were fed a high cholesterol diet they exhibited almost perfect down regulation of endogenous cholesterol synthesis. Fractional absorption of cholesterol was unchanged, fecal neutral steroid excretion was increased, and fecal bile acid output remained constant upon shifting from a low to high cholesterol intake. The overall result of these metabolic changes was a 50% reduction in the rate of cholesterol synthesis. The authors calculate that the compensatory response accounted for all but 0.2 mg/kg/day of the increment in absorbed cholesterol, which may have accumulated in body tissues during the study. Similar precision in feedback regulation of cholesterol metabolism has been reported for New Guinea Highlanders, who have a higher fractional absorption of dietary cholesterol and a lower basal cholesterol synthesis rate than the Tarahumara Indians, who were able to reduce endogenous cholesterol synthesis by 68% when given a dietary cholesterol challenge.[34] These cross-cultural studies suggest that the ability to regulate cholesterol synthesis exists in other ethnic populations and is apparently independent of cultural dietary patterns.

There is no evidence that dietary cholesterol contributes to the risk of gallstone formation[35] even though a primary compensatory response to a high cholesterol intake is increased biliary re-excretion of the absorbed sterol.[27-30] Supersaturation of bile with cholesterol has not been found in patients fed high cholesterol diets.[35]

Sterol balance studies carried out in infants and young children have shown that the rate of whole body cholesterol synthesis changes during the first few months of life, from a relatively high level (17 mg/kg/day) to a value not significantly different from that found in adults.[36-40] The biological causes of this initially high cholesterol synthesis rate and its subsequent decrease after the first months of life are completely unknown. The existence of feedback responses to dietary cholesterol have been demonstrated in young children.[37,39] Martin and Nestel[39] studied children between the ages of 5 to 18 years and found that when dietary cholesterol intake was increased 450 mg/day, cholesterol balance decreased in most of the children. The data indicated that the metabolic heterogeneity of responses to a dietary cholesterol challenge in children was similar to that found in adults. In a similar study, Nestel et al.[37] tested the response of ten infants, between 3 and 16 months of age, on a low and high cholesterol intake and found that net sterol balance fell substantially during the high dietary cholesterol period. It should be noted, however, that sterol balance studies in growing infants and children are not carried out in the metabolic steady state since body weights increase throughout the study and net influx of cholesterol occurs throughout the growth period in order to satisfy tissue needs for cholesterol in membranes. Thus, all values for sterol synthesis rates in growing children represent a minimal estimate since the quantitative significance and variations of the cholesterol influx can only be approximated.

2. Fat Quality

The quality of dietary fat, P:S ratio (ratio of polyunsaturated to saturated fat), has profound effects on plasma cholesterol levels in humans, and numerous studies have attempted to define the metabolic effects of a change in fat quality on whole body sterol metabolism. Initial studies suggested that a shift from a saturated- to polyunsaturated-fat containing diet resulted in a significant increase in fecal steroid excretion and that this increased excretion could quantitatively account for the magnitude of the decrease in plasma cholesterol levels.[41-43] Subsequent studies by Grundy and Ahrens[44] refuted this concept of increased excretion of steroid due to a high P:S diet, and provided evidence that exchanging dietary fat quality from a low to high P:S ratio had no effect on total fecal steroid excretion once a new steady state had been achieved. Similar findings of the lack of effect of polyunsaturated fat diets on fecal steroid excretion have been reported.[45,46]

In part these conflicting findings have been resolved by the report of Grundy[47] that a patient's type of hyperlipidemia accounts for whether or not an increase in P:S ratio results in an increased fecal sterol excretion. The Grundy study demonstrated that hypertriglyceridemic patients who have elevated rates of endogenous cholesterol synthesis significantly increase fecal sterol excretion upon intake of a high P:S diet. A second possible explanation for the conflicting reports regarding increases in fecal steroid excretion during intake of a polyunsaturated fat diet may be due to the time interval between the change in dietary fat and the establishment of a new steady state in plasma cholesterol levels and fecal steroid excretion. The available data would suggest an increased fecal excretion of neutral steroids does occur immediately following a shift of dietary fat quality, but this increased fecal excretion, if it occurs at all, appears to be a transient phase which is found during the establishment of a lower plasma cholesterol level. The currently available data indicate that polyunsaturated fat in the diet has no effect on the rate of whole body cholesterol synthesis.[48]

The intake of high polyunsaturated fat diets has been shown to increase biliary cholesterol saturation in some patients,[47] primarily in those individuals who exhibit an increased fecal neutral steroid excretion when shifted to a high P:S diet. The evidence is far from conclusive regarding the generality of this finding and, therefore, the effect of polyunsaturated fat diets on biliary composition remains in doubt.[35]

3. Fat Quantity

Any attempt to define the effect of total fat calories on whole body cholesterol metabolism must be interpreted with caution, since the shift in fat calories must, by necessity, be offset by a corresponding shift in carbohydrate intake in order to maintain a eucaloric, weight-maintaining diet (metabolic steady state); thus, the quandry of determining whether the change in fat calories or carbohdyrate calories caused the observed changes. It is necessary in this context to consider the relative contributions of these two nutrients to the diet and to view any change in sterol metabolism as a result of the shift in the fat:carbohydrate ratio. Three studies have investigated the effects of fat:carbohydrate quantity on sterol balance in man, and indicate that a shift in fat/carbohydrate calories results in variable effects on whole body cholesterol synthesis rates. Schreibman and Ahrens[49] reported that a shift from 70 to 20% of calories from polyunsaturated fat caused a significant increase in fecal steroid excretion in 4 of 10 patients, a decrease in 4, and no change in 2; 2 patients exhibited a significant increase in bile acid excretion when shifted from a high fat to high carbohydrate diet.

In a similar study, Cummings et al.[50] reported that shifting patients from a low fat (21% of calories) to a high fat (48%) diet caused a twofold increase in fecal bile acid output in all subjects studied. In contrast, Andersen and Hellstrom[51] reported that patients on 60.4% of calories from fat vs. 27.8% of calories did not change total sterol balance but did shift fecal steroid output with an increase in fecal bile acid output and a corresponding decrease in fecal neutral steroid excretion. The decrease in fecal neutral steroid output was consistent with the finding of reduced cholesterol concentrations in duodenal bile of patients on the low fat diet.[51]

The data are extremely inconsistent on the effects of fat quantity on whole body cholesterol metabolism and in part relate to a number of variables: dietary fat quality used in the diets, the types of hyperlipidemic patients under study, and the use of liquid-formula vs. solid-food diets. Both Schreibman and Ahrens[49] and Andersen and Hellstrom[51] reported increased plasma triglyceride levels in all patients shifted from a high fat to low fat diet, which may account for the increase in sterol balance found by Schreibman and Ahrens in some patients[49] since hypertriglyceridemia is related to an increased production of cholesterol. At the present time it is not possible to define what effect a shift in the ratio of fat/carbohydrate calories has on whole body cholesterol metabolism.

4. Other Fats

Sitosterol —Studies by Grundy et al.[26] originally demonstrated that the plant sterol sitosterol, given at a dosage of 5.5 to 11.0 g/day, inhibited dietary cholesterol absorption in man and resulted in an increase in endogenous cholesterol synthesis. Subsequent studies by Lees et al.[52] provided evidence that maximal plasma cholesterol lowering could be achieved by daily administration of 3 g/day of a tall oil suspension of sitosterol. At this level of dietary sitosterol intake exogenous cholesterol absorption decreased by 50% and endogenous cholesterol excretion doubled, indicative of a reduced absorption of endogenous biliary cholesterol.

A recent report by Mattson et al.[53] demonstrated that the large quantities of sitosterol used in previous studies were not necessary to achieve an inhibition of cholesterol absorption. Feeding patients a diet containing 500 mg/day of cholesterol plus 1 g sitosterol or 2 g sitosterol oleate caused a 42 and 35% reduction in cholesterol absorption, respectively. The decreased cholesterol absorption was accompanied by a decrease in plasma cholesterol levels. The sitosterol content of the average diet approximates 250 mg/day and at this level would be expected to have little effect on whole body cholesterol metabolism.

Sucrose polyester — The fat substitute, sucrose polyester (SPE), is composed of hexa-, hepta-, and octaesters of sucrose which are not hydrolyzed by pancreatic lipase and not absorbed. Crouse and Grundy[54] studied the effect of SPE on cholesterol absorption and synthesis in a group of obese patients during weight loss (a nonsteady-state situation) and showed that SPE feeding reduced plasma cholesterol levels by 7%, decreased cholesterol absorption by an average of 55%, and increased the fecal excretion of both neutral and acidic sterols. The use of SPE as a plasma cholesterol lowering agent and as a fat substitute for weight reduction has another advantage in that SPE does not increase the cholesterol saturation of gallbladder bile and will not increase the risk of gallstone formation associated with some cholesterol lowering modalities.

C. Dietary Protein

A limited number of studies investigating the effect of vegetable vs. animal dietary protein on whole body cholesterol metabolism have been reported in humans. These studies have consistently shown that substitution of soy protein for casein, or addition of soy-containing foods to the basal diet, have no effect on cholesterol or bile acid synthesis, even under conditions where plasma cholesterol levels are reduced by the change in source of dietary protein.[55-58] Studies by Calvert et al.[56] tested the hypothesis that the saponin content of vegetable protein may be involved in intestinal binding of bile acids and their increased excretion. Their results demonstrated that altering the saponin intake five-fold had no effect on fecal bile acid excretion. The available data indicate that dietary protein has no effect on cholesterol or bile acid synthesis rates in man; and as such, alterations in whole body cholesterol metabolism cannot account for their reported hypocholesterolemic effect.

D. Dietary Carbohydrates

As noted above, it is difficult to determine the effect of the amount of dietary carbohydrates on cholesterol metabolism since a decrease in carbohydrate intake is equivalent to an increase in fat intake. The reader is referred to the section above on dietary fat quantity.

There is conflicting experimental evidence linking sucrose intake with an increased risk of gallstone formation due to increased biliary cholesterol saturation. Cahlin et al.[59] reported increased biliary saturation with cholesterol when patients were fed high as compared to low refined carbohydrates; however, this finding was not corroborated by the findings of Thornton et al.[60] and Werner et al.[61] who found no effect of sucrose on biliary composition in patients with radiolucent gallstones. The evidence would suggest that intake of refined carbohydrates in a eucaloric diet that maintains ideal body weight does not increase bile saturation or gallstone formation.

The effects of alcohol intake on whole body cholesterol metabolism have been studied in a small number of patients[62,63] and the data indicate that alcohol intake has no effect on the absorption of dietary cholesterol or on cholesterol and bile acid synthesis rates. The studies by Crouse and Grundy[63] demonstrated that alcohol intake did not affect the composition of bile even though very low density lipoprotein (VLDL) triglyceride and high density lipoprotein (HDL) cholesterol levels increased during the alcohol intake period.

E. Dietary Fiber

In vitro bile acid binding capacity of nondigestible plant carbohydrates is a well-documented property of fiber.[64,65] Metabolic studies suggest that water insoluble plant fibers are relatively ineffective in lowering plasma cholesterol levels while the water soluble fibers do have cholesterol lowering properties.[64,65] Two natural gel-forming fibers, pectin and guar gum, increase fecal bile acid excretion in man when fed at levels of 15 to 50 g/day.[66,67] Cellulose, but not methyl cellulose, also reduces plasma cholesterol levels, apparently by increasing fecal bile acid excretion.[68,69] Other fibers which reduce plasma cholesterol and increase fecal bile acid excretion include Bengal gram,[70] oat bran,[71,72] and corn bran.[73] Studies by Judd and Truswell[74] found no significant differences in fecal bile acid excretion between high and low methoxyl pectins. No dietary fiber tested to date has increased fecal neutral steroid excretion, yet guar gum administration does reduce dietary cholesterol absorption.[75]

While some fibers reduce plasma cholesterol levels and increase fecal bile acid excretion, a number of dietary fibers reduce plasma cholesterols without affecting fecal steroid output. Gum arabic,[76] cooked wheat bran,[77] and bean supplement[72] reduce plasma cholesterol levels yet have no effect on fecal bile acid excretion. In a comparative study of oat-bran- and bean-supplemented diets, Anderson et al.[72] reported that both high fiber sources reduced plasma cholesterol levels; however, oat bran caused a 65% increase in fecal bile acids and bean supplement resulted in a 30% decrease in fecal acidic sterols.

The data suggest that water soluble fiber in the diet can effectively reduce plasma cholesterol levels, in part due to their ability to bind bile acids in the gastrointestinal tract. The plasma cholesterol lowering mechanism is similar to that of the hypolipidemic drug cholestryramine, yet this must be only a partial explanation since increased fecal acidic sterol excretion is not a consistent finding for all plasma cholesterol lowering fibers and, on a comparative basis to the drug cholestyramine, the increment in fecal bile acid excretion is not sufficient to explain the magnitude of the plasma cholesterol lowering. Dietary fibers can have a significant effect on whole body cholesterol metabolism but its plasma cholesterol lowering mechanism(s) remain to be fully elucidated.

Epidemiological evidence suggests a relationship between a low fiber intake and increased incidence of gallstones. Consumption of fiber-rich bran diets may reduce the cholesterol saturation of bile in patients with gallstones[78,79] but has not been shown to alter biliary composition in normal subjects who do not have saturated bile and are free of gallstones.[80,81] In those situations where fiber diets have reduced biliary cholesterol saturation, it has been accompanied by a change in bile acid composition and a reduction in the proportion of secondary bile acids found in bile. Studies by Huijbregts et al.[82] on the effects of feeding wheat bran on biliary lipid composition demonstrated that 0.5 g/kg/day of wheat bran, which lowered plasma cholesterol levels, did not change either biliary lipid and bile acid composition; bile acid synthesis rates and pool sizes; or total fecal excretion of neutral and acidic steroids. The authors conclude that wheat bran is not effective in lowering biliary cholesterol saturation in normal males.[82] The evidence suggests that dietary fiber has little effect on biliary cholesterol saturation in individuals without existing saturated bile, but may have value in the treatment of patients with lithogenic bile and thus at high risk for gallstones.

F. Other Dietary Factors

Ascorbic acid — Studies by Duane and Hutton[83] on the effect of short-term subclinical ascorbic acid deficiency near the ascorbutic range demonstrated that vitamin C had no effect on plasma lipoprotein cholesterol levels, biliary lipid composition, bile acid kinetics, or sterol balance.

IV. CONCLUSIONS AND SUMMARY

Sterol balance measurements of whole body cholesterol homeostasis have made possible the characterization of the interactions of a number of nutrients with whole body cholesterol metabolism in man. Studies carried out in laboratories around the world have shown that most components of the diet can alter plasma cholesterol levels and whole body cholesterol metabolism. When sterol balance measurements are combined with the studies of in vivo lipoprotein metabolism, a clearer understanding of the interrelationships between the metabolism of the lipoproteins (the carrier) and cholesterol (the load in the carriers) as related to cardiovascular diseases and gallstone formation can be obtained. More importantly, the data from such studies can be used to determine the efficacy of interventions designed to reduce plasma and biliary cholesterol levels and their associated risk of atherosclerosis and cholelithiasis. We can now ask not only whether a dietary treatment lowers plasma cholesterol levels, but where does the cholesterol go when it leaves the plasma compartment and what metabolic changes in cholesterol homeostasis are taking place.

In trying to understand the relationship between plasma cholesterol levels and whole body cholesterol metabolism, one of the most striking observations is that plasma cholesterol levels are in no way related quantitatively to the key parameters of endogenous sterol metabolism. Whole body cholesterol synthesis rates are the same for patients with a cholesterol level of 150 mg/dℓ as for those with levels of 350 mg/dℓ; 11 mg/kg/day. In the steady-state situation, under which most studies are carried out, the rates

Table 2
CHOLESTEROL METABOLISM

Dietary Factor	Absorption	Synthesis	Catabolism	Excretion	Tissue flux
Calories	—	↑	—	↑	↑
Cholesterol	—	↓	↑	↑	?
PUFA	—	—	—	—, ↑	↑
Sitosterol	↓	↑	—	↑	?
SPE	↓	↑	—	↑	?
Vegetable protein	—	—	—	—	?
CHO	—	↑	↑	↑	?
EtOH	—	—	—	—	?
Fiber	↓	—	—	—	?

Note: PUFA, polyunsaturated fat; SPE, sucrose polyester; CHO, carbohydrate calories; EtOH, ethanol.

of inputs to and outputs from the cholesterol pool are the same in everyone; only the actual pool sizes (primarily the plasma and total exchangeable pools) differ. An important, and as yet unresolved, question is whether metabolic or genetic processes determine the size of the plasma and whole body cholesterol pools and when in the course of development is it determined. This aspect of whole body cholesterol metabolism, and the role that dietary factors may play in determining plasma cholesterol levels remain one of the major unresolved problems in our quest to understand the regulation of cholesterol metabolism in man.

What dietary factor has the greatest impact on whole body cholesterol metabolism? The evidence indicates that total calories and body weight have the largest single effect on cholesterol synthesis, pool size, and biliary saturation, in addition to an increased incidence of hyperlipidemia (Table 2). Obesity and a hypercaloric intake exert more influence on cholesterol metabolism and pool size than any single, or combination, of dietary constituents, and as such represent the major determinants of sterol metabolism in the majority of individuals. To reduce hyperlipidemia, an expanded cholesterol pool and biliary saturation with cholesterol, the most effective intervention is weight reduction and maintenance of an ideal body weight. No single dietary intervention has the potential to be as effective.

Obesity has been shown to be an independent risk factor for cardiovascular disease[84] and recent studies have shown that the distribution of fat deposits may be a better predictor of cardiovascular disease and death than the degree of adiposity.[85,86] The recognition of "androgenic obesity" as a risk factor for cardiovascular disease[87] in men and women, and the high prevalence of obesity in our society, necessitates an increased public awareness of the hazards of being overweight. The relationship between altered cholesterol metabolism and increased heart disease risk in obese individuals, and the fact that this altered metabolic pattern can be reversed by weight reduction, should provide a strong incentive for the patient at risk for cardiovascular disease to decrease caloric intake and increase caloric expenditure through exercise.

As noted above, newborn infants have elevated rates of whole body cholesterol synthesis which decreases after the first 6 months of life to a level indentical to that found in adults. A recent report by Einarsson et al.[88] has shown that there are changes in biliary secretion of cholesterol and bile acid synthesis with age. In a group of males and females who were not obese and were free of gallstones, these investigators found a positive correlation between age and cholesterol saturation of bile and cholesterol secretion rates, and a negative correlation with bile acid synthesis and the size of the bile acid pool. The combination of increased biliary cholesterol secretion and decreased bile acid synthesis with age may explain the increased risk of gallstone formation with age.

One final point of importance in attempting to understand the interplay between nutrients and whole body cholesterol metabolism is the ever present complication of the metabolic heterogeneity of humans, and their lack of a predictable response to a given intervention. No doubt much of the conflicting effects found using the same dietary intervention can be ascribed to this individuality of control mechanisms and compensatory responses.[89] Generalizations run the risk of oversimplification and of not providing the individual patient with the individualized care he or she requires. As has been seen in this review, the cholesterol homeostatic response achieved by any dietary manipulation can be dependent upon the patient's type of hyperlipidemia, adiposity, and biliary composition; and as such, interventions to reduce cardiovascular disease or gallstone risk must be based on the combination of our curent understanding of the generalities of cholesterol metabolism and the idiosyncrasies of the metabolism of the individual.

ACKNOWLEDGMENT

It is with great pleasure that I dedicate this chapter to E. H. Ahrens, Jr. M.D., Professor, The Rockefeller University, whose contributions to the development and application of sterol balance techniques have directly and indirectly, through the continued use of sterol balance techniques by many of those trained in his laboratory, provided much of the basis for our current understanding of whole body sterol metabolism and the role of diet in cholesterol homeostasis. This chapter was written in part under support of Public Health Service Grant HL 35417.

REFERENCES

1. Miettinen, T. A., Ahrens, E. H., Jr., and Grundy, S. M., Quantitative isolation and gas-liquid chromatographic analysis of total dietary and fecal neutral steroids, *J. Lipid Res.*, 6, 411, 1965.
2. Grundy, S. M., Ahrens, E. H., Jr., and Miettinen, T. A., Quantitative isolation and gas-liquid chromatographic analysis of fecal bile acids, *J. Lipid Res.*, 6, 397, 1965.
3. Grundy, S. M., Ahrens, E. H., Jr., and Salen, G., Dietary B-sitosterol as an internal standard to correct for cholesterol losses in sterol balance measurements, *J. Lipid Res.*, 9, 374, 1968.
4. Davignon, J., Simmonds, W. J., and Ahrens, E. H., Jr., Usefulness of chromic oxide as an internal standard for balance studies in formula-fed patients and for assessment of colonic function, *J. Clin. Invest.*, 47, 127, 1968.
5. Grundy, S. M. and Ahrens, E. H., Jr., Measurements of cholesterol turnover, synthesis, and absorption in man, carried out by isotope kinetics and sterol balance measurements, *J. Lipid Res.*, 10, 91, 1969.
6. Smith, F. R., Dell, R. B., Noble, R. P., and Goodman, DeW. S., Parameters of the three-pool model of the turnover of plasma cholesterol in normal and hyperlipidemic humans, *J. Clin. Invest.*, 57, 137, 1976.
7. Samuel, P. and Lieberman, S., Improved estimation of body masses and turnover of cholesterol by input-output analysis, J. Lipid Res., 14, 189, 1973.
8. Samuel, P., Lieberman, S., and Ahrens, E. H., Jr., Comparison of cholesterol turnover by sterol balance and input-output analysis, and a shortened way to estimate total exchangeable mass of cholesterol by the combination of the two methods, *J. Lipid Res.*, 19, 94, 1978.
9. Borgstrom, B., Quantification of cholesterol absorption in man by fecal analysis after the feeding of a single isotope-labeled meal, *J. Lipid Res.*, 10, 331, 1969.

10. Quintao, E., Grundy, S. M., and Ahrens, E. H., Jr., An evaluation of four methods for measuring cholesterol absorption by the intestine in man, *J. Lipid Res.,* 12, 221, 1971.
11. Samuel, P., Crouse, J. R., and Ahrens, E. H., Jr., Evaluation of an isotope ratio method for measurement of cholesterol absorption in man, *J. Lipid Res.,* 19, 82, 1978.
12. Crouse, J. R. and Grundy, S. M., Evaluation of a continuous isotope feeding method for measurement of cholesterol absorption in man, *J. Lipid Res.,* 19, 967, 1978.
13. Grundy, S. M. and Mok, H. Y. I., Determination of absorption in man by intestinal perfusion, *J. Lipid Res.,* 18, 263, 1977.
14. Samuel, P., McNamara, D. J., Ahrens, E. H., Jr., Crouse, J. R., and Parker, T., Further validation of the plasma isotope ratio method for measurement of cholesterol absorption in man, *J. Lipid Res.,* 23, 480, 1982.
15. Samuel, P. and McNamara, D. J., Differential absorption of exogenous and endogenous cholesterol in man, *J. Lipid Res.,* 24, 265, 1983.
16. McNamara, D. J., Prediction of plasma cholesterol responses to dietary cholesterol, *Am. J. Clin. Nutr.,* 41, 657, 1985.
17. Nikkari, T., Schreibman, P. H., and Ahrens, E. H., Jr., Isotope kinetics of human skin cholesterol secretion, *J. Exp. Med.,* 141, 620, 1975.
18. Crouse, J. R., Grundy, S. M., and Ahrens, E. H., Jr., Cholesterol distribution in the bulk tissues of man: variations with age, *J. Clin. Invest.,* 51, 1292, 1972.
19. Nestel, P. J., Whyte, H. M., and Goodman, DeW. S., Distribution and turnover of cholesterol in humans, *J. Clin. Invest.,* 48, 982, 1969.
20. Nestel, P. J., Schreibman, P. H., and Ahrens, E. H., Jr., Cholesterol metabolism in human obesity, *J. Clin. Invest.,* 52, 2389, 1973.
21. Miettinen, T. A., Cholesterol production in obesity, *Circulation,* 44, 842, 1971.
22. Miettinen, T. A., Fecal steroid excretion during weight reduction in obese patients with hyperlipidemia, *Clin. Chim. Acta,* 19, 341, 1968.
23. Schreibman, P. H. and Dell, R. B., Human adipocyte cholesterol. Concentration, localization, synthesis and turnover, *J. Clin. Invest.,* 55, 986, 1975.
24. Bennion, L. J. and Grundy, S. M., Effects of obesity and caloric intake on biliary lipid metabolism in man, *J. Clin. Invest.,* 56, 996-1011, 1975.
25. Goodman, DeW. S., Smith, F. R., Seplowitz, A. H., Ramakrishnan, R., and Dell, R. B., Prediction of the parameters of whole body cholesterol metabolism in humans, *J. Lipid Res.,* 21, 699, 1980.
26. Grundy, S. M., Ahrens, E. H., Jr., and Davigon, J., The interaction of cholesterol absorption and cholesterol synthesis in man, *J. Lipid Res.,* 10, 304, 1969.
27. Quintao, E., Grundy, S. M., and Ahrens, E. H., Jr., Effects of dietary cholesterol on the regulation of total body cholesterol in man, *J. Lipid Res.,* 12, 233, 1971.
28. Quintao, E. C. R., Brumer, S., and Stechhahn, K., Tissue storage and control of cholesterol metabolism in man on high cholesterol diets, *Atherosclerosis,* 26, 297, 1977.
29. Maranhao, R. C. and Quintao, E. C. R., Long term steroid metabolism balance studies in subjects on cholesterol-free and cholesterol-rich diets: comparison between normal and hypercholesterolemic individuals, *J. Lipid Res.,* 24, 167, 1983.
30. Nestel, P. J. and Poyser, A., Changes in cholesterol synthesis and excretion when cholesterol intake is increased, *Metabolism,* 25, 1591, 1976.
31. Mistry, P., Miller, N. E., Laker, M., Hazzard, W. R., and Lewis, B., Individual variation in the effects of dietary cholesterol on plasma lipoproteins and cellular cholesterol homeostasis in man, *J. Clin. Invest.,* 67, 493, 1981.
32. Parker, T. S., McNamara, D. J., Brown, C., Garrigan, O., Kolb, R., Batwin, H., and Ahrens, E. H., Jr., Mevalonic acid in human plasma: relationship of concentration and circadian rhythm to cholesterol synthesis rates in man, *Proc. Natl. Acad. Sci. U.S.A.,* 79, 3037, 1982.
33. McMurry, M. P., Connor, W. E., Lin, D. S., Cerqueira, M. T., and Connor, S. L., The absorption of cholesterol and the sterol balance in the Tarahumara Indians of Mexico fed cholesterol free and high cholesterol diets, *Am. J. Clin. Nutr.,* 41, 1289, 1985.
34. Whyte, M., Nestel, P., and MacGregor, A., Cholesterol metabolism in Papua New Guineans, *Eur. J. Clin. Invest.,* 7, 53, 1977.
35. Bennion, L. J. and Grundy, S. M., Risk factors for the development of cholelithiasis in man. *N. Engl. J. Med.,* 299, 1221, 1978.
36. Potter, J. M. and Nestel, P. J., Greater bile acid excretion with soy bean than with cow milk in infants, *Am. J. Clin. Nutr.,* 29, 546, 1976.
37. Nestel, P. J., Poyser, A., and Boulton, T. J. C., Changes in cholesterol metabolism in infants in response to dietary cholesterol and fat, *Am. J. Clin. Nutr.,* 32, 2177, 1979.
38. Huang, C. T. L., Rodriguez, J. T., Woodward, W. E., and Nichols, B. L., Comparison of patterns of fecal bile acid and neutral sterol between children and adults, *Am. J. Clin. Nutr.,* 29, 1196, 1979.

39. Martin, G. M. and Nestel, P., Changes in cholesterol metabolism with dietary cholesterol in children with familial hypercholesterolaemia, *Clin. Sci.*, 56, 377, 1979.

40. Zavoral, J. H., Laine, D. C., Bale, L. K., Wellik, D. L., Ellefson, Kuba, K., Krivit, W., and Kottke, B. A., Cholesterol excretion studies in familial hypercholesterolemic children and their normolipidemic siblings, *Am. J. Clin. Nutr.*, 35, 1360, 1982.

41. Moore, R. B., Anderson, J. T., Taylor, H. L., Keys, A., and Frantz, I. D., Jr., Effect of dietary fat on the fecal excretion of cholesterol products in man, *J. Clin. Invest.*, 47, 1517, 1968.

42. Connor, W. E., Witiak, D. T., Stone, D. B., and Armstrong, M. L., Cholesterol balance and fecal neutral steroid and bile acid excretion in normal men fed dietary fats of different fatty acid composition, *J. Clin. Invest.*, 48, 1363, 1969.

43. Nestel, P. J., Havenstein, N., Scott, T. W., and Cook, L. J., Polyunsaturated ruminant fats and cholesterol metabolism in man, *Aust. N.Z. J. Med.*, 4, 497, 1974.

44. Grundy, S. M. and Ahrens, E. H., Jr., The effects of unsaturated dietary fats on absorption, excretion, synthesis and distribution of cholesterol in man, *J. Clin. Invest.*, 49, 1135, 1970.

45. Nestel, P. J. and Homma, Y., Effect of dietary polyunsaturated pork on plasma lipid and sterol excretion in man, *Lipids*, 11, 42, 1976.

46. Shepherd, J., Packard, C. J., Grundy, S. M., Yeshurun, D., Gotto, A. M., Jr., and Tauton, O. D., Effects of saturated and polyunsaturated fat diets on the chemical composition and metabolism of low density lipoproteins in man, *J. Lipid Res.*, 21, 91, 1980.

47. Grundy, S. M., Effects of polyunsaturated fats on lipid metabolism in patients with hypertriglyceridemia, *J. Clin. Invest.*, 55, 269, 1975.

48. Goodnight, S. H., Jr., Harris, W. S., Connor, W. E., and Illingworth, D. R., Polyunsaturated fatty acids, hyperlipidemia, and thrombosis, *Arteriosclerosis*, 2, 87, 1982.

49. Schreibman, P. H. and Ahrens, E. H., Jr., Sterol balance in hyperlipidemic patients after dietary exchange of carbohydrate for fat, *J. Lipid Res.*, 17, 97, 1976.

50. Cummings, J. H., Wiggins, H. S., Jenkins, D. J. A., Houston, H., Jivraj, T., Drasar, B. S., and Hill, M. J., Influence of diets high and low in animal fat on bowel habit, gastrointestinal transit time, fecal microflora, bile acid, and fat excretion, *J. Clin. Invest.*, 69, 953, 1978.

51. Andersen, E. and Hellstrom, K., Influence of fat-rich versus carbohydrate-rich diets on bile acid kinetics, biliary lipids, and net steroid balance in hyperlipidemic subjects, *Metabolism*, 29, 400, 1980.

52. Lees, A. M., Mok, H. Y. I., Lees, R. S., McClusky, M. A., and Grundy, S. M., Plant sterols as cholesterol-lowering agents: clinical trials in patients with hypercholesterolemia and studies of sterol balance, *Atherosclerosis*, 28, 325, 1984.

53. Mattson, F. H., Grundy, S. M., and Crouse, J. R., Optimizing the effect of plant sterols on cholesterol absorption in man, *Am. J. Clin. Nutr.*, 35, 697, 1982.

54. Crouse, J. R. and Grundy, S. M., Effects of sucrose polyester on cholesterol metabolism in man, *Metabolism*, 28, 994, 1979.

55. Potter, J. D., Illman, R. J., Calvert, G. D., Oakenfull, D.G., and Topping, D. L., Soya saponins, plasma lipids, lipoproteins and fecal bile acids: a double blind crossover study, *Nutr. Rep. Int.*, 22, 521, 1980.

56. Calvert, G. D., Blight, L., Illman, R. J., Topping, D. L., and Potter, J. D., A trial of the effects of soya-bean flour and soya-bean saponins on plasma lipids, faecal bile acids and neutral sterols in hypercholesterolemic men, *Br. J. Nutr.*, 45, 277, 1981.

57. Fumagalli, R., Soleri, L., Farina, R., Musanti, R., Mantero, O., Noseda, G., Gatti, E., and Sirtori, C. R., Fecal cholesterol excretion studies in Type II hypercholesterolemic patients treated with the soybean protein diet, *Atherosclerosis*, 42, 341, 1982.

58. Grundy, S. M. and Abrams, J. J., Comparison of actions of soy protein and casein on metabolism of plasma lipoproteins and cholesterol in humans, *Am. J. Clin. Nutr.*, 38, 245, 1983.

59. Cahlin, E., Jonsson, J., Nilsson, S., and Schersten, T., Biliary lipid composition in normolipidemic and prebeta hyperlipidemic gallstone patients. Influence of sucrose feeding of the patient on the biliary lipid composition, *Scand. J. Gastroenterol.*, 8, 449, 1973.

60. Thornton, J. R., Emmett, P. M., and Heaton, K. W., Diet and gallstones: effects of refined and unrefined carbohydrate diets on bile saturation and bile acid metabolism, *Gut*, 2, 2, 1983.

61. Werner, D., Emmett, P. M., and Heaton, K. W., Effects of dietary sucrose on factors influencing cholesterol gallstone formation, *Br. Med. J.*, 25, 269, 1984.

62. Nestel, P. J., Simons, L. A., and Homma, Y., Effects of alcohol on bile acid and cholesterol metabolism, *Am. J. Clin. Nutr.*, 29, 1007, 1976.

63. Crouse, J. R. and Grundy, S. M., Effects of alcohol on plasma lipoproteins and cholesterol and triglyceride metabolism in man, *J. Lipid Res.*, 25, 486, 1984.

64. Huang, C. T. L., Gopalakrishna, G. S., and Nichols, B. L., Fiber, intestinal sterols, and colon cancer, *Am. J. Clin. Nutr.*, 31, 516, 1978.

65. Anderson, J. W. and Chen, W-J. L., Plant fiber. Carbohydrate and lipid metabolism, *Am. J. Clin. Nutr.*, 32, 346, 1979.

66. Kay, R. M. and Truswell, A. S., Effect of citrus pectin on blood lipids and fecal steroid excretion in man, *Am. J. Clin. Nutr.*, 30, 171, 1977.

67. Miettinen, T. A. and Tarpila, S., Effect of pectin on serum cholesterol, fecal bile acids and biliary lipids in normolipidemic and hyperlipidemic individuals, *Clin. Chim. Acta*, 79, 471, 1977.

68. Forman, D. T., Garvin, J. E., Forenster, J. E., and Taylor, C. B., Increased excretion of fecal bile acids by an oral hydrophilic colloid, *Proc. Soc. Exp. Biol. Med.*, 127, 1060, 1968.

69. Stanley, M. M., Paul, D., Gacke, D., and Murphy, J., Effects of cholestyramine, metamucil and cellulose on fecal bile salt excretion in man, *Gastroenterology*, 65, 889, 1973.

70. Mathur, K. S., Khan, M.A., and Sharma, R. D., Hypocholesterolemic effect of Bengal gram: a long-term study in man, *Br. Med. J.*, 1, 30, 1968.

71. Kirby, R. W., Anderson, J. W., Seilig, B., Rees, E. D., Chen, W-J. L., Miller, R. E., and Kay, R. M., Oat-bran intake selectively lowers serum low-density lipoprotein cholesterol concentrations of hypercholesterolemic men. *Am. J. Clin. Nutr.*, 34, 824, 1981.

72. Anderson, J. W., Story, L., Sieling, B., Chen, W-J. L., Petro, M. S., and Story, J., Hypocholesterolemic effects of oat-bran or bean intake for hypercholesterolemic men, *Am. J. Clin. Nutr.*, 40, 1146, 1984.

73. Bell, E. W., Emken, E. A., Klevay, L. M., and Sandstead, H. H., Effects of dietary fiber from wheat, corn, and soy hull bran on excretion of fecal bile acids in humans, *Am. J. Clin. Nutr.*, 34, 1071, 1981.

74. Judd, P. A. and Truswell, A. S., Comparison of the effects of high- and low-methoxyl pectins on blood and fecal lipids in man, *Br. J. Nutr.*, 48, 451, 1982.

75. Simons, L. A., Gayst, S., Balasubramaniam, S., and Ruys, J., Long-term treatment of hypercholesterolaemia with a new palatable formulation of guar gum, *Atherosclerosis*, 45, 101, 1982.

76. Ross, A. H. M., Eastwood, M. A., Brydon, W. G., Anderson, J. R., and Anderson, D. M. W., A study of the effects of dietary gum arabic in humans, *Am. J. Clin. Nutr.*, 37, 368, 1983.

77. Ross, J. K. and Leklem, J. E., The effects of dietary wheat bran on human fecal parameters and neutral and acidic steroid excretion, *Nutr. Rep. Int.*, 28, 1271, 1983.

78. Pomare, E. W., Heaton, K. W., Low-Beer, T. S., and Espiner, H. J., The effect of wheat bran upon bile salt metabolism and upon the lipid composition of bile in gallstone patients, *Am. J. Dig. Dis.*, 21, 521, 1976.

79. McDougall, R. M., Yakymshyn, L., Walker, K., and Thurston, O. G., Effect of wheat bran on serum lipoproteins and biliary lipids, *Can. J. Surg.*, 21, 433, 1978.

80. Watts, J. McK., Jablonski, L., and Toouli, J., The effect of added bran to the diet on the saturation of bile in people without gallstones, *Am. J. Surg.*, 135, 321, 1978.

81. Wicks, A. C. B. Yeates, J., and Heaton, K. W., Bran and bile: time-course of changes in normal young men given a standard dose, *Scand. J. Gastroenterol.*, 13, 289, 1978.

82. Huijbregts, A. W. M., Van Berge-Henegouwen, G. P., Hectors, M. P. C., Van Schaik, A., and Van der Werf, S. D. J., Effects of a standardized wheat bran preparation on biliary lipid composition and bile acid metabolism in young healthy males, *Eur. J. Clin. Invest.*, 10, 451, 1980.

83. Duane, W. C. and Hutton, S. W., Lack of effect of experimental ascorbic acid deficiency on bile acid metabolism, sterol balance, and biliary lipid metabolism in man, *J. Lipid Res.*, 24, 1186, 1983.

84. Hubert, H. B., Feinleib, M., McNamara, P. M., and Castelli, W. P., Obesity as an independent risk factor for cardiovascular disease: a 26-year follow-up of participants in the Framingham Heart Study, *Circulation*, 67, 968, 1983.

85. Larsson, B., Svardsudd, K., Welin, L., Wilhelmsen, L., Bjorntorp. P., and Tibblin, G., Abdominal adipose tissue distribution, obesity, and risk of cardiovascular disease and death: 13-year follow up of participants in the study of men born in 1913, *Br. Med. J.*, 288, 1401, 1984.

86. Bjorntorp, P., Hazards in subgroups of human obesity, *Eur. J. Clin. Invest.*, 14, 239, 1984.

87. Ahrens, E. H., Jr., Obesity and coronary heart disease. New dimensions, *Arteriosclerosis*, 4, 177, 1984.

88. Einarsson, K., Nilsell, K., Leijd, B., and Angelin, B., Influence of age on secretion of cholesterol and synthesis of bile acids by the liver, *N. Engl. J. Med.*, 313, 277, 1985.

89. McNamara, D. J., Diet and hyperlipidemia. A justifiable debate, *Arch. Intern. Med.*, 142, 1121, 1982.

Chapter 5

THE ROLE OF OXIDIZED LIPIDS IN HEART DISEASE AND AGING

Terrance L. Smith and Fred A. Kummerow

TABLE OF CONTENTS

I. INTRODUCTION

Cardiovascular disease is the largest single cause of death in the U.S., accounting for 45 to 50% of all deaths.[1] About 75% of all deaths from cardiovascular disease are due to heart disease, the most common feature of which is some form of atherosclerosis. Typically, atherosclerosis involves a thickening of the aortic intima (see Figure 1) and deposition of plaque resulting in a lesion. This lesion is filled with lipid, particularly cholesterol and cholesterol ester, connective tissue, macrophages and foam cells, smooth muscle cells, and frequently in advanced stages, calcium.

At present the most widely accepted theory of atherogenesis points to cholesterol as the most important agent in the initiation of lesion formation. It is thought that hypercholesterolemia causes an increase in the membrane cholesterol content of endothelial cells resulting in cellular damage, which allows low density lipoprotein (LDL) to accumulate in the intima.[2,3] This is followed by a sequence of events involving loss of endothelial integrity, further accumulation of LDL, stimulation of smooth muscle cell (SMC) growth, and accumulation of macrophages.[4] The accumulation of lipid in the intima eventually leads to the engorgement of macrophages and possibly SMC with cholesterol ester and triggers their conversion to foam cells.[5] The consequence of these events is the formation of an atherosclerotic lesion.

Such a central role for cholesterol in heart disease is generally referred to as the "lipid hypothesis". Not everyone agrees with this viewpoint, and the debate it has generated has frequently been acrimonious. Harper[6] lists the main arguments in favor of and opposing the lipid hypothesis, and these are tabulated here (Table 1). Epidemiological studies and their statistical evaluation are frequent sources of controversy. The relationship between serum cholesterol and heart disease often breaks down, particularly for women and those over 65. Likewise, a large portion of those experiencing heart attack in the Framingham study had "safe" levels of serum cholesterol (below 235 mg%).[7] Criticism of experiments in which laboratory animals are induced to develop atherosclerosis by feeding cholesterol is based on the amount of dietary cholesterol needed to produce the desired effect. Typically, as much as 10 times the level of cholesterol found in the American diet must be fed before atherogenesis in laboratory animals occurs. Other experiments have thrown doubt on the atherogenicity of cholesterol by showing that initiation of the disease is due to contaminants in U.S.P. cholesterol.[8-10] These contaminants were found to be auto-oxidation products of cholesterol. 25-Hydroxycholesterol was the most atherogenic and the major oxidation product present. Feeding of pure cholesterol, free of auto-oxidation products, did not cause the initiation of atherosclerosis in test animals. The use of familial hypercholesterolemia as a model system is open to criticism since it is an abnormal state. It should probably be viewed as a distinct disease and not typical of otherwise normal patients with heart disease.

It is our opinion that while cholesterol may predispose persons with familial hyperlipidemia to atherosclerosis, it is not by itself capable of accounting for atherosclerosis in the general population. While lipid peroxidation products are not the only possible secondary agents in atherogenesis, there is reason to believe they are an important factor. Lipid peroxidation products are present in heart disease patients; they are capable of causing injury to cells and cause morphological changes to endothelial cells similar to those seen in the early stages of atherosclerosis. After reviewing the ways lipid peroxidation may be involved in atherosclerosis, we will describe a model of how peroxidation could be atherogenic and the possible relations between aging, lipid peroxidation, and heart disease.

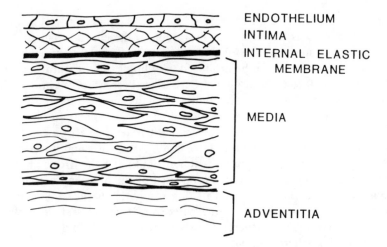

FIGURE 1.   The aorta wall; Endothelium — cell monolayer that coats the inner wall of the arteries and veins; Intima — connective tissue between the endothelium and internal elastic membrane. It is this area that is invaded by LDL and cells during formation of a lesion. Internal elastic membrane — the small pore size of this membrane traps LDL in the intima; Media — mostly smooth muscle cells; Involved in vessel contraction; Adventitia — outer layer of smooth muscle cells; Carries vasculature to nourish the outer portion of the wall; Inner portions draw nourishment from the lumen.

Table 1
THE LIPID HYPOTHESIS CONTROVERSY

Pro	Con
A positive statistical correlation is observed between cholesterol and fat consumption and heart disease	There are many expectations to these correlations, and other factors correlate as well
There is a statistically significant change in the serum lipid level and heart disease rate of animals on high lipid diets	Unrealistically high lipid levels are required in the diet to produce an effect
There is a correlation between serum cholesterol levels and the rate of heart disease in humans	The relation is not a direct one and breaks down for women and persons over 65
Persons with familial hyperlipidemia have high incidence of heart disease	This is probably a special case and does not relate to the general population
Dietary manipulation can reduce serum cholesterol 10—15%	Clinical trials show little effect on heart disease rate even with a 10% decrease in serum cholesterol

II. INCIDENCE OF LIPID PEROXIDATION IN HEART DISEASE SUBJECTS

A. Tissue and Lesions

Atherosclerotic tissues and lesions have been examined for the presence of lipid peroxidation products, and both ceroid and lipid peroxide have been found. Ceroid is derived from lipids; it binds lipid stains but is insoluble in lipid solvents. It is naturally fluorescent and in general seems to be identical with the pigments isolated from other tissues and referred to as age pigment, lipofuscin, or lipochrome. The lipids found in ceroid include cholesterol and cholesterol esters, triglycerides, and phospholipids. While a ceroid-like material can be produced with lipids only, natural ceroid has been reported to contain 30 to 60% protein.[11] Ceroid has been observed in the atherosclerotic arteries of a range of animals including humans, dogs, rats, and rabbits.[12,13] A direct correlation has also been observed between ceroid content and intimal thickening, which is considered to be an early stage in atherogenesis. However, the consensus has been that ceroid only accumulates later in atherosclerosis and is due to secondary degeneration. It may act as a fibrotic agent contributing to the irreversibility of atherosclerotic lesions. This role of ceroid is supported by the observation that injection of synthetic material into the aortic wall of dog results in the development of fibrosis within 4 weeks.[14] Low sensitivity in the detection of ceroid and the general use of animals in advanced stages of atherosclerosis make it difficult to determine if ceroid is involved in initiating atherosclerosis.

It is also possible and even likely that ceroid precursors such as lipoperoxide are the true threat in atherogenesis. Healthy aortas are found to contain no lipoperoxide, while diseased tissues contain amounts that correlate with the extent of tissue damage.[15] Lipoperoxides are easily generated as artifacts in the extraction process,[16] but diseased tissues extracted under conditions which prevent artifact formation have also been shown to contain lipoperoxide.[17] Cholesterol esters of hydroxy fatty acids have been isolated from atherosclerotic plaques, and it is suggested that their most likely source is the degradation of lipid peroxides.[18,19] The lipid in atherosclerotic plaques is derived from serum lipids particularly LDL and very low density lipoprotein (VLDL). Attempts to determine the extent of peroxidation of lipoproteins extracted from arterial walls have not been made, but the presence of peroxidation can be demonstrated.

Aortic wall tissue from rabbits fed a cholesterol-rich diet for 4 weeks showed elevated levels of lipid peroxidation (as TBA reactive products).[20] There were also elevated levels of glutathione disulfide in the tissue. Glutathione disulfide is produced when hydrogen peroxide is reduced to water by glutathione peroxidase. In humans, the electrophoretic mobility of LDL isolated from atherosclerotic areas was greater than that of serum LDL.[21,22] This difference in mobility is typical of peroxidation modified LDL, as described later in this review.

B. Serum Peroxidation

Elevated serum lipoprotein levels are associated with a risk of heart disease. In particular, LDL is thought to be atherogenic and high density lipoprotein (HDL) a protective factor against atherosclerosis. Diabetics have a high risk of heart disease, elevated serum lipids, and elevated serum lipid peroxide levels.

Fractionation of the lipoproteins reveals that LDL in both normal and diabetic humans contains the major concentration of the lipid peroxides (Table 2).[23] However, the increase in serum lipid peroxidation among diabetics is mostly due to elevated levels in the HDL fraction. The significance of this is not clear but may represent accumulation of lipid by the proposed lipid scavenging activity of HDL. Diabetics free of vascular disease have serum lipid peroxidation levels similar to nondiabetics, while diabetics with vascular disease have nearly twice the peroxide level.[24] Unfortunately, it is not clear from this experiment whether this represents a causative effect or is a result of heart disease. Subfractionation of lipoprotein classes into constituent lipid classes and determination of peroxidation content show variation in the distribution of peroxides between both lipoprotein classes and normal vs. diabetic.[23] In the normal population, LDL and VLDL triglyceride contained the highest levels of peroxidation, while in the

Table 2
LIPID PEROXIDE LEVELS OF SERUM
LIPOPROTEIN FRACTIONS OF NORMAL
AND DIABETIC SUBJECTS

	n	VLDL	LDL	HDL
			Lipid peroxides[a]	
Normal	32	0.64 ± 0.30	1.18 ± 0.33	0.68 ± 0.16
Diabetic	31	0.68 ± 0.34	1.26 ± 0.35	1.07 ± 0.40[b]

[a] Lipid peroxide level is expressed in terms of malondialde-
    hyde (nmol/m*l* serum). Mean ± SD is given.
[b] $p < 0.001$.

From Nishigaki, I., Hagihara, M., Tsunekawa, H., Maseki,
M., and Yagi, K., *Biochem. Med.*, 25, 378, 1981. With permission.

diabetics all LDL components were peroxidized, and LDL cholesterol peroxidation
and HDL phospholipid peroxidation increased. The association of lipid peroxidation
with serum triglyceride and phospholipid has also been observed in restricted ovulator
chickens,[25] which readily develop atherosclerosis.

III. CELL INJURY BY LIPID PEROXIDATION

Polyunsaturated fatty acids undergo peroxidation by a free radical reaction. This
produces lipid peroxy radicals that can initiate further peroxidation and lipid peroxides
which may degrade to malondialdehyde. Malondialdehyde reacts with aminophospholipids or proteins to form a Schiff's base of the general structure R−N=C−C=C−N−R,
where R represents an amine group.[26] This compound is autofluorescent, and its measurement has been used as an assay for lipid peroxidation. The loss of unsaturated acyl
chains and of the aminophospholipids due to peroxidation would be expected to alter
the lipid membrane properties. An increase in the gel-like character of the membrane
has been noted and attributed to a loss of unsaturation.[27] Electron spin resonance
studies indicate that the loss of fluidity is primarily due to alterations in the transmembrane fluidity gradient at about the 10th to 12th carbon.[28,29] This can be interpreted as
the loss of unsaturation, which woul have a major effect on that region, or as a cross-
linking of acyl chains via peroxide linkages. The loss of phosphatidylethanolamine
(PE) to form Schiff's base results in an altered membrane structure.[30] At physiological
temperatures and pH, PE prefers the hexagonal (H_{II}) phase to the bilayer phase. Peroxidation resulted in destabilization of the H_{II} and formation of a bilayer even though
74% of the PE had a free amino group. Phosphatidylethanolamine was found to be
more sensitive to peroxidation than phosphatidylcholine, possibly due to PEs greater
unsaturation. While it is not firmly established that nonbilayer membrane structures
are physiologically relevant, this does demonstrate a means by which the disruption of
membranes may occur with peroxidation. The membrane of most cells has been shown
to possess an asymmetry between the leaflets, which probably is of importance to cellular function.[31] The erythrocyte has a particularly well-characterized membrane asymmetry of the aminophospholipids. When exposed to malondialdehyde, either generated
in the membrane or added exogenously, this asymmetry is broken down.[32] This loss of
asymmetry may be due to the reaction of malondialdehyde with either phosphatidylethanolamine or spectrin. Peroxidation has also been found to increase the rate of trans-

Table 3

ENZYME INACTIVATION BY LIPID
PEROXIDATION

Tissue	Enzyme	Site of action	Ref.
Liver	Cytochrome P-450	Protein	39
			40
Liver	Glucose-6-phosphatase	Lipid	41
			40
Heart	NADH oxidase	Lipid	42
Mitochondria	NADH cytochrome c reductase	Lipid	
	Succinate oxidase	Lipid	
	Succinate cytochrome c reductase	Lipid	
	Succinate dehydrogenase	Protein	
Adrenal gland	Monooxygenase	Lipid	43
	Cytochrome P-450	Protein	
	NADPH cytochrome c reductase	Protein	
	NADPH cytochrome c reductase	Protein	
Unspecified microsome	Ca ATPase	Protein	44
Liver microsomes	Ca ATPase	Protein	45

bilayer movement of phosphatidylcholine.[33,34] Lipid vesicles were found to have no detectible transbilayer motion until lipid peroxidation reached a critical level after 5 to 7 days. While the precise role of nonbilayer membrane structures and bilayer asymmetry is not known, they are likely of physiological importance, and the ability of lipid peroxidation to alter these structures illustrates their damaging potential.

Most membrane proteins have been shown to have a lipid requirement. For most, this is a nonspecific requirement for a lipid environment.[35] However, some have a specific phospholipid head group requirement of which β-hydroxybutyrate dehydrogenase is the best characterized. An absolute requirement for phosphatidylcholine (PC) has been demonstrated,[36] but maximum activity is only achieved by a mixture of phosphatidylcholine, phosphatidylethanolamine, and cardiolipin.[37] Cytochrome oxidase activity in reconstituted vesicles requires both phosphatidylcholine and phosphatidylethanolamine.[38] Neither lipid by itself was able to stimulate the activity of the enzyme due to leakiness of the vesicles. Tightly coupled vesicles and hence maximal activity were only obtained with mixtures of PC and PE. The two differently shaped molecules together are able to seal the protein into the membrane. The loss of PE through peroxidation could conceivably cause adverse changes in enzymatic activity.

Lipid peroxidation effects on proteins also result in loss of enzymatic activity (Table 3). Cytochrome P-450, which is involved in the liver with xenobiotic detoxification, provides an example. When presented with carbon tetrachloride, its detoxification attempt results in the formation of a CCl_3 radical which can either instigate the peroxidation of lipids or destroy the cytochrome P-450. Liver cells exposed to carbon tetrachloride produce lipid peroxidation products and lose cytochrome P-450 activity. The peroxidative reaction subsides when 85 to 95% of the cytochrome P-450 is inactivated. Glucose-6-phosphatase activity is reduced in response to peroxidation, but this is thought to be due to the loss of required lipid environment. In this case the loss of activity due to peroxidation is very similar to that seen when lipid is removed by detergent treatment or phospholipase, and exogenously added malondialdehyde had no effect on glucose-6-phosphatase activity. Lipid peroxidation of mitochondria resulted in a loss of the ability to conduct respiration, with the electron transport chain affected at several sites due to the loss of lipid environment. The calcium pump activity of microsomes has been completely destroyed by as little as 5 μg MDA/g equivalent microsome. This amount of peroxidation is much less than that frequently reported for in vitro peroxidation of microsomes and demonstrates the sensitivity of this protein. When the pump was protected with 5 mM ATP, 12 μg MDA/gram equivalent microsomes were required to reduce activity to 3% of controls.

Malondialdehyde may also induce the polymerization of proteins as has been documented in the erythrocyte. SDS gel electrophoresis shows a loss of staining intensity of most protein bands and the concomitant appearance of a large molecular weight band.[46-48] One investigator has also observed a low molecular weight band which may be the result of protein cleavage.[47]

Lipid membranes containing peroxidation products have been shown to have increased permeability to ions and biological molecules. Above a threshold level of 5% peroxidation, release of glucose from liposomes is proportional to the extent of peroxidation.[49] Oxidation also renders lipid bilayers permeable to ions including potassium,[50,51] chromate,[52] and calcium.[53,54] The increase in permeability does not seem to be due to the slight change in phase transition temperature resulting from loss of unsaturated fatty acids. Studies on mixed phosphatidylcholines indicate that 5.6% mixtures do induce phase separation but only over a 1° range.[55] An alternate explanation would be that lipid peroxides form transient channels for the passage of ions, and the 5% minimum represents a level required for the statistical formation of peroxide clusters.[56,57]

Several lipid peroxidation products have been tested to determine their activity as ionophores in lipid vesicles. Water soluble products including malondialdehyde were released from peroxidizing membranes, but these products had no effect on the permeability of fresh vesicles to which they were added.[58] Lysophosphatidic acid is a known surfactant and a product of lipid peroxidation which remains in the membrane. Incorporation of lysophosphatidylcholine in vesicles resulted in a slightly permeable membrane. However, the permeability was not as great as vesicles peroxidized *in situ* to the same content of lysophosphatidylcholine.[59] Unpublished results from our laboratory indicate that the Schiff base product of peroxidation is completely incapable of causing membrane permeability.[131] The oxidized sterol, 25-hydroxycholesterol, is an effective permeability agent for a number of divalent and monovalent ions.[54] Lipid peroxides have also been shown to be effective in promoting ion permeability of bilayers.[56,131]

IV. ENDOTHELIAL CELLS, PEROXIDATION, AND ATHEROSCLEROSIS

Damage to the aortic endothelial cell layer is one of the earlier events in atherogenesis. Normal endothelium is composed of flat, elongated cells which tightly abut one another. Injured cells become cuboidal in shape, develop blebs, and may contract from adjacent cells depending on the extent of injury.[60,61] Early theories of endothelial injury suggested that loss of cell attachment occurred quickly,[4] but more recent studies suggest denudation is a later event.[62] Monkeys fed an atherogenic diet developed foam cells after only 1 month during which time the endothelial layer remained intact. Only after 4 months did the cells shrink from their junctional complexes, and after 5 months desquamation began to occur. This correlates well with earlier work done in rabbits fed a hypercholesterolemic diet.[63] After 3 weeks on this diet, alterations in endothelial morphology were noted, including irregular shape and increased permeability to silver stain. However, the lesions remained covered by endothelium even after 6 months of hypercholesterolemia. While injury sufficient to cause cell death is probably not the earliest event of atherogenesis, it is evident that a less extensive injury to the endothelium is an important factor in atherogenesis. The ability of cells to transport Evan's Blue dye attached to albumin into the subendothelial space is a means of localizing injured cells. Areas of the aorta which collect the dye are covered by endothelial cells with an injured morphology, a reduced glycolcalyx, and larger numbers of lysosomes.[60] The endothelial layer acts as a selective permeability barrier maintaining an intimal concentration of albumin about half that of the serum and a concentration of LDL about twice that of the serum.[64] An increased transport of serum components into the intima, originally demonstrated by the Evans Blue technique, has been quantitated in E.B. Smith's laboratory. Areas under gelatinous and transitional lesions were found to have LDL concentrations of 145 and 185%, respectively, of the normal intimal LDL concentration.[65] Studies using diabetic rats indicate that the rate of albumin transfer into aorta is greater in diabetic than control animals.[66] Diabetes is a major risk factor for heart disease, and it is estimated that 80% of diabetics die of complications from atherosclerosis. The rate of transcytosis of albumin by endothelial cells in tissue culture was affected by free fatty acids in the medium.[67] At fatty acid-to-albumin ratios greater than 1, the rate of transcellular movement of albumin was increased. Linoleic acid had a greater effect than oleic acid, and a significant alteration in the fatty acid composition of the cellular membrane was observed. The mechanism by which the observed increase in albumin transfer occurred is not known but may be due to changes in membrane fluidity, as speculated by Hennig et al.,[67] or due to peroxidation. Most of the fatty acid taken up by the cells was recovered from phospholipid and triglyceride, leaving very small amounts available for peroxidation. These small amounts, however, may be sufficient to cause the observed effect. A model of how this could occur will be discussed later in this chapter.

Lipid peroxidation is capable of causing endothelial damage of the type under discussion. Injection of linoleic acid hydroperoxides into rabbits resulted in a rapid alteration in endothelial cell morphology, which was similar to that seen in early stages of atherosclerosis.[68] Arachidonic acid caused lesion formation in brain arteriols,[69] but this damage was prevented by antioxidants. The generation of hydrogen peroxide in endothelial cells by xanthine oxidase results in increased permeability to potassium ions, altered prostaglandin synthesis, and release of cytosolic purines.[70] Of particular note is the observation that these effects occurred at hydrogen peroxide levels 30-fold less than those causing cell death.

V. PEROXIDATION AND OTHER COMPONENTS IMPLICATED IN ATHEROSCLEROSIS

A. Platelets

Platelets do not adhere to normal endothelium. If the integrity of the endothelium is compromised they will adhere to the exposed collagen. This is an important step in the endothelial injury hypothesis of atherogenesis as platelets release a potent growth factor (PDGF). This growth factor stimulates the proliferation of smooth muscle cells and encourages their invasion of the intima.[71,72] Activated platelets also released malondialdehyde as a by-product of thromboxane synthesis.[73] The ability of malondialdehyde produced in this manner to adversely affect endothelial cells has not been shown but could represent a source of cellular injury. Such an event might assume great significance if the endothelial cells were altered to allow the adherance of platelets as has been shown to occur in virally transformed endothelial cells.[74]

B. Neutrophiles

Neutrophiles undergo a transient attachment to the endothelium. This attachment is greatly augmented by inflammation. Stimulated neutrophiles are capable of killing endothelial cells in tissue culture by the release of hydrogen peroxide[75,76] or can cause the release of unlysed cells by proteolytic activity.[77] The importance of this activity in atherogenesis is not known but could represent yet another source of endothelial injury through peroxidation.

C. LDL Cytotoxicity

As mentioned earlier, LDL and HDL are thought to have opposing activities with LDL being atherogenic. The LDL fraction of serum lipoproteins is found to contain the highest level of lipid peroxidation.[23,78] The accumulation of peroxidation products in LDL results in a modification of the LDL. Modified LDL has a greater negative charge and moves farther on an electrophoresis gel.[79] The increase in negative charge is due to the reaction of malondialdehyde with the lysine residues of apolipoprotein B.[80,81] The change in charge is evidently responsible for recognition of modified LDL by the nonregulated "scavanger" pathway of monocytes and endothelial cells.[82] When less than 15% of the exposed lysines were modified, the LDL was taken up by the normal LDL receptor, while at higher levels of modification the LDL was taken up by the "scavenger" receptor.[80]

The modification of LDL by lipid peroxidation is responsible for LDL cytotoxicity toward endothelial cells in tissue culture.[83,84] While the modification of lysine residues is responsible for the uptake of LDL by the nonregulated receptor, the cytotoxic compound is a chloroform-methanol extractable molecule, and protection from peroxidative reactions prevented cytotoxicity.[85] Only one peroxidation product in LDL has been identified and it is 25-hydroxycholesterol.[86]

HDL is thought to be protective against atherosclerosis and has been found also to protect tissue culture cells from LDL toxicity.[83,87] The mode of action of this protective effect is not known, but it was suggested by Henriksen[83] that reduced binding of LDL to receptor-independent sites could explain the observations. Such an effect of HDL on fibroblasts binding of LDL has already been observed.[88] A similar receptor has since been shown to be present in endothelial cells.[82] Confluent endothelial cells have relatively few LDL receptors but readily take up modified LDL by the receptor independent pathways. It has not yet been demonstrated that HDL reduces the binding of LDL to these endothelial receptors, but these experiments do suggest a biochemical reason for the epidemiological evidence relating to HDL:LDL ratios and heart disease. They also suggest that in the absence of peroxidation modified LDL, lower amounts of HDL may not necessarily represent an elevated risk of heart disease.

Generally experiments on LDL cytotoxicity have used in vitro modified LDL or LDL which has become modified through peroxidation in the isolation process. The effect of hyperlipidemic LDL on smooth muscle cells shows it to have a mitotic effect.[89] We have not been able to locate similar studies done on endothelial cells. Also these cytotoxic studies have been designed to look for extensive cellular injury and death. The effects proposed in this review would be due to milder, nonlethal injury resulting in abnormal cellular activity.

D. Macrophages

Most, if not all, "foam cells" found in the intima are now recognized as being derived from macrophages.[90] The foamy appearance of these cells is due to a massive accumulation of lipid (especially cholesterol ester) in the cell in the form of lipid droplets. Lipoproteins enter macrophages by a receptor-mediated endocytosis and the cholesterol then enters a cycle of ester hydrolysis and re-esterification.[5,80,92] In this cycle, the linoleate ester of cholesterol found in the serum is replaced by an oleate ester which enters storage. If cholesterol acceptors such as HDL are available, then the cholesteryl oleate is hydrolyzed and cholesterol is excreted to the acceptor. The receptor for LDL endocytosis is strongly regulated by intracellular cholesterol concentration. Consequently, it is impossible to convert macrophages to foam cells when exposed only to normal LDL. Modified LDL enters the macrophage by the receptor-independent pathway which is not subject to feedback regulation.[5,91,92] Therefore, macrophages presented with modified LDL ingest it unchecked and are readily converted to foam cells. Modifying treatments of LDL causing recognition by this receptor include acetylation, maleylation, succinylation,[93] acetoacetylation,[94] and malondialdehyde treatment.[79,93] Of these, malondialdehyde treatment is of greatest interest since there is some evidence that LDL can be modified in this manner in vivo, and such LDL has been isolated from humans as discussed earlier. Macrophages also accumulate cholesterol through a receptor for very low density lipoprotein (β-VLDL).[95] This lipoprotein is found in hypercholesterolemic animals and differs from normal VLDL by having less triglyceride and more cholesterol ester in the core and by having reduced amounts of apo C.[5] Of particular interest to us is the implication that if modified LDL or β-VLDL is not present, foam cells will not be formed.

E. Smooth Muscle Cells

Smooth muscle cells may be involved in lesion formation by proliferating into the intima. These cells are stimulated in their growth by factors derived from both monocytes and platelets. Subfractions of LDL may also be mitogenic toward smooth muscle cells.[96] Large LDL (molecular weight $> 3.0 \times 10^6$) from normolipidemic or hyperlipidemic monkeys but not smaller LDLs were found to have this effect. The mechanism for mitotic activity of these LDLs is not known.

VI. LIPID PEROXIDATION AND ATHEROGENESIS

A. A Model of Atherogenesis

Thus far in this chapter it has been demonstrated that lipid peroxidation can be detected at higher levels in subjects with atherosclerosis and that diabetics, who are at risk toward heart disease, also have elevated levels of peroxidation. We have also discussed the cell-damaging effects of lipid peroxidation and peroxidation products. Central to our model is the role of calcium as an intracellular messenger.

Intracellular calcium concentrations are on the order of 10^{-6} M while the serum calcium concentration is 10^{-3} M. The maintenance of this 1000-fold difference depends on limited entry and active removal of calcium ions.[97] The cellular lipid membrane is very impermeable to ions, allowing a highly controlled calcium influx. An influx of calcium occurs in response to hormones, growth factors, chemotactic substances, and eicosanoids. The increase of intracellular calcium concentration functions with cAMP as a secondary messenger for extracellular signals. The removal of calcium involves sodium-calcium exchange protein, an ATP requiring calcium pump, and the binding of free calcium by intracellular molecules. Calcium ATPase may either pump calcium out of the cell or into mitochondria and endoplasmic reticulum where it is sequestered and is available for release upon proper stimulation. Endocytosis[98] and exocytosis[99] are both sensitive to cellular calcium levels, with increased calcium concentration increasing the rate of endo- and exocytosis. It might therefore be expected that an increasingly leaky endothelial membrane would result in increased transcytoic movement of serum components to the intima. Phospholipase A is also activated by calcium, and the re-

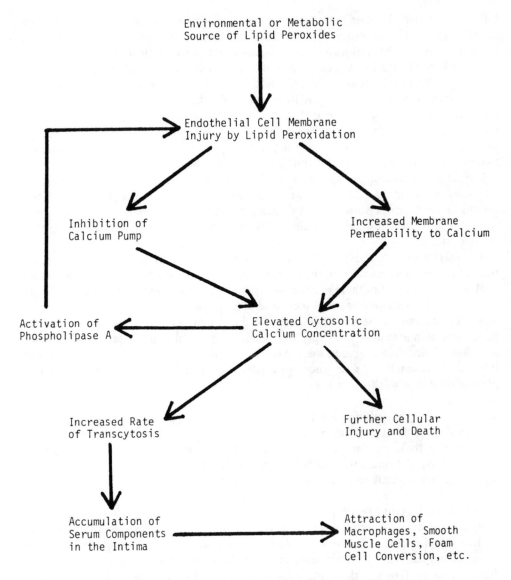

FIGURE 2.   Possible sequence of events in atherogenesis by lipid peroxidation.

sulting activity will further increase membrane damage through generation of lyso-phospholipids and increased peroxidation.[100,101] A vicious cycle may then ensue, with calcium levels eventually reaching toxic concentrations.[102,103]

Accumulation of peroxidation products in the plasma membrane of endothelial cells will result in an alteration in the physical properties including the increased permeability to calcium (Figure 2). Unpublished data from our laboratory[132] indicates that of the three major peroxidative products (Schiff's base, malondialdehyde, lipid peroxide), only lipid peroxide causes phosphatidylcholine liposomes to become permeable to calcium. The in vivo source of these lipid peroxides might be environmental or metabolic. Metabolic sources would include the modification of LDL by endothelial cells, prostaglandin synthesis, metabolism of free fatty acids released by lipoprotein lipase, or derangement of electron transport chains. Environmental factors might include ingestion of preformed peroxidation products or attempts at detoxification of xenobiotics.

The accumulation of lipid peroxidation products, in addition to allowing a greater influx of calcium, inhibits the activity of the ATP-dependent calcium pump. Consequently, as more calcium begins to enter the cell, the ability to remove calcium is also impaired. The resulting elevation in cytosolic calcium will activate phospholipase A, which in turn increases the membrane damage by accumulation of lysophospholipids and enhanced peroxidation. This could lead to a quick cascade of damage, killing the cell. Areas that are dyed by Evans Blue in vivo do show higher numbers of dead endothelial cells than other areas of the aorta.[60] Death of cells may be avoided if peroxidative rates are low enough that the damage can be contained by normal cell regeneration and repair. This may provide a partial explanation for the frequent statistical anomalies in the correlation of serum lipid levels and heart disease.

Hyperlipidemia may provide a larger vehicle for the transport of peroxidation products (i.e., in modified LDL), but the actual level of peroxidation may be low. Based on this model, such persons would be expected to have a low incidence of heart disease while persons with low serum lipid levels that are highly peroxidized would be at greater risk.

The elevated calcium level in the cytosol is expected to increase the rate of transcytosis of serum components into the intima. Not only will there be an increase in intimal LDL concentration, but there may be an enrichment in modified LDL since endothelial cells, like macrophages, have an increased affinity for acetylated LDL.[82] Monocytes would be attracted by serum lipoproteins in the intima, and events from this point on likely follow the sequence already derived by others: macrophages ingest excessive amounts of modified LDL and are converted to foam cells. A lesion forms as extracellular lipid accumulates, and smooth muscle cells are stimulated by macrophage or platelet derived growth factors.

B. Source of Lipid Peroxidation Products

If lipid peroxidation is an important factor in atherosclerosis, then the possible sources of peroxidation must be determined. While considerable research on peroxidation in biological membranes has been conducted, the events which occur in vivo are still not clear. Nevertheless, several possible sources can be mentioned.

1. Arachidonic Acid Metabolism

Arachidonic acid is a major substrate for the production of prostaglandins. Malondialdehyde is produced in the arachidonate oxygenation pathway in platelets leading to thromboxane B_2.[104,105] Since malondialdehyde has not proved a potent cellular initiator of peroxidation in the studies discussed above, the importance of this source of peroxidation remains to be determined. Another feature of arachidonic acid prostaglandin metabolism is the production of hydro- and endoperoxides by lipoxygenase and cyclooxygenase. These lipid peroxides are both intermediates in and regulators of prostaglandin synthesis and have short lifetimes.[106] Their contribution to peroxidative cell injury is therefore probably small, unless the supply of glutathion peroxidase and glutathion transferase is interrupted.

2. Modification of LDL

Endothelial and smooth muscle cells in tissue culture modify LDL.[107,108] Free radical scavengers or metal chelators eliminate the peroxidative effect and support the idea that the effect is a free radical type of reaction. A considerable degree of conversion of LDL phosphatidylcholine to lysophosphatidylcholine was observed, which was also inhibited by antioxidants. It is not clear whether this also occurs in vivo. Since antioxidants such as BHT are able to prevent endothelial cell modification of LDL, a sufficient vitamin E status in the animal may prevent its occurrence.

3. Lipoprotein Lipase Generation of Free Fatty Acids

Lipoprotein lipase (LPL) has recently been located on the endothelium of bovine aorta.[109] This enzyme releases free fatty acids from chylomicrons and VLDL, apparently to allow its movement into and across the endothelium.[110] Zilversmit[111] has suggested that LPL and hypertriglyceridemia may result in the generation of harmful levels of free fatty acids. Free fatty acid levels of greater than 30 μM inhibited most cells in tissue culture. Smooth muscle cells in tissue culture underwent lipid peroxidation when exposed to free fatty acids.[112] Inhibitor studies showed that the peroxidation was not occurring in the medium, nor by a variety of intracellular pathways. All of the data suggests induction of the peroxisomal enzyme systems by the free fatty acids and the consequent production of hydrogen peroxide. Peroxisomal proliferation has been associated with lipid peroxidation in other studies as well. Lipofuscin granules frequently are found to be associated with peroxisomes,[113] and peroxisomal proliferators such as methyl clofenapate also cause a concomitant increase in cellular peroxidation.[114] While this is a very intriguing pathway, its importance to atherosclerosis remains unknown.

4. Detoxification and Peroxidation

Hepatic attempts at detoxification can result in lipid peroxidation. Carbon tetrachloride toxicity arises in such a manner. Cytochrome P-450 acting on carbon tetrachloride produces a CCl_3 radical, setting in motion peroxidative events which both destroy the cytochrome and peroxidize nearby lipids.[39,115,116] Peroxidizing liver microsomes are known to produce water soluble products which are capable of crossing a dialysis membrane and thereby damaging target cells.[117] These long-lived, water-soluble products could enter the blood stream, causing damage to lipoproteins, erythrocytes, or endothelial cells. Alternatively, since the liver is a major site of lipoprotein metabolism, it is possible that peroxidative reactions originating from the cytochromes might affect lipoproteins as well. Some support for this comes from the observations that human patients with liver diseases (hepatitis, cirrhosis, or fatty liver) also have elevated serum lipid levels.[118] Whether or not this will lead to endothelial injury is not known.

5. Metabolic Production of Free Radicals

Enzymatic reactions other than drug hydroxylation may produce free radicals. In some cases this is a desired product, as in the use of superoxide by phagocytes to kill engulfed bacteria.[119] Oxidative enzymes such as xanthine oxidase have been used in vitro to produce free radicals for peroxidation reactions.[120,121] This type of enzymatic formation of radicals probably occurs only under unusual circumstances, as intermediate products are normally directly transferred to the next enzyme in the series. Only when this chain is disrupted is it possible to initiate radical formation.

6. Ingestion of Preformed Lipid Peroxides

The high temperatures involved in deep fat frying can lead to breakdown of the fat and accumulation of lipid peroxidation products.[122] Alexander[123] reviewed the effects of thermally oxidized fats on rat heart, liver, and kidney. All of these tissues showed abnormalities with heart damage occurring exclusively in the blood vessel walls. In a recent study rats fed thermally oxidized frying oil were found to have accumulated lipid peroxidation products in the liver.[124] Dietary oxidized cholesterol has already been mentioned as being implicated in atherogenesis.[10] In both of these cases the dietary level must be high to see an effect on the animals and may not represent typical intake in humans.

C. Cellular Protection from Peroxidation

Cells and tissues are well supplied with defenses against peroxidative damage in the

Table 4
SERUM LIPID PEROXIDE
LEVELS OF NORMAL
SUBJECTS

Age (years)	Lipid peroxide level	
	Male	Female
0—10	1.86 ± 0.60	2.04 ± 0.48
11—20	2.64 ± 0.60	2.64 ± 0.54
21—30	3.14 ± 0.56	2.98 ± 0.50
31—40	3.76 ± 0.52	3.06 ± 0.50
41—50	3.94 ± 0.60	3.16 ± 0.54
51—60	3.92 ± 0.92	3.30 ± 0.74
61—70	3.94 ± 0.70	3.46 ± 0.72
71—	3.76 ± 0.76	3.30 ± 0.78

Note: Lipid peroxide level is expressed in terms of malondialdehyde (nmol/m*l* of serum). Mean ± SD.

From Yagi, K., Ed., *Lipid Peroxides in Biology and Medicine,* Academic Press, New York, 1982, 223. With permission.

form of superoxide dismutase, catalase, the glutathione oxidase system, and vitamin E.[125] These enzymes provide protection by reducing superoxide ion to water and by converting free fatty acid lipid peroxides to the corresponding fatty alcohol. For peroxidation to occur and cause cellular damage, these defenses must be either overwhelmed or circumvented. That this does occur to some extent is indicated by the presence of lipid peroxides in the blood and tissue of both healthy and diseased subjects.

VII. AGING, HEART DISEASE, AND LIPID PEROXIDATION

Heart disease is accepted as a disease of aging whose initiation may begin in very young children. Thickening of the intima to the same extent of that found in adults is often noted within the first few months after birth.[126] Coronary fatty streaks are found in 10-year-old children, and their number tends to increase until age 30. By age 20 fibrous plaques are found, and they increase in number for the remaining lifespan. There is a sharp increase in the amount of fibrous plaque at 30 years coincident with the decrease in fatty streak.[127] It is this relationship which suggests that fatty streaks are converted into fibrous plaques, although this progression is questioned by those who observe that aortic fatty streaks, unlike coronary fatty streaks, do not always form at sites sensitive to advanced lesion formation.[128] By the 40- to 50-year period advanced lesions form, presumably from fibrous plaques, and clinical symptoms begin to occur. Differences with age have been observed in lipoprotein levels, and these also could have an effect on the progression of heart disease.[129] The plasma cholesterol increases in both men and women between the ages of 15 and 55. In both men and women LDL cholesterol increases and HDL cholesterol decreases at puberty. However, male HDL cholesterol then remains constant while female HDL cholesterol rises until menopause.

It is interesting to note that serum lipid peroxidation also increases with age (Table 4).[130] Peroxidation levels increase through the 41- to 50-year age group for males and the 61- to 70-year group for females. In addition, the overall mean is higher for men than for women. The reason for this increase is not known, nor is its relation to heart disease and age-related changes in lipoprotein metabolism known.

VIII. CONCLUSION

In this discussion we have presented the hypothesis that lipid peroxidation plays a part in the initiation of heart disease. Lipid peroxidation is found to be associated with heart disease both in the diseased tissue and the blood plasma. Diabetes, a risk factor for heart disease, has been found to be accompanied by elevated serum levels of lipid peroxidation. It has been demonstrated that lipid peroxidation products are damaging to the cell and can initiate a sequence of events leading to an atherosclerotic lesion. Of particular importance to this scheme is the effect of lipid peroxidation products on the calcium permeability of lipid membranes and the conversion of macrophages to foam cells by peroxide modified LDL. All of the individual steps proposed for this model have been demonstrated by various researchers. However, it remains to be seen if these events occur in vivo to an extent sufficient to contribute to heart disease. The source of lipid peroxidation in the body is another unanswered question, as are the factors affecting the levels of peroxidation in the plasma.

It is apparent that our understanding of the very earliest steps in atherogenesis is meager. The model presented here suggests areas where profitable studies might be done.

REFERENCES

1. Omran, A. R., Epidemiologic transition in the U.S.: the health factor in population change, *Population Bulletin*, 32, No. 2, Population Reference Bureau, Washington, D.C., 1977.
2. Jackson, R. L. and Gotto, A. M., Jr., Hypothesis concerning membrane structure, cholesterol, and atherogenesis, *Atheroscler. Rev.*, 1, 1, 1976.
3. Papahadjopoulos, D., Cholesterol and cell membrane function: a hypothesis concerning the etiology of atherosclerosis, *J. Theor. Biol.*, 43, 329, 1974.
4. Ross, R. and Harker, L., Hyperlipidemia and atherosclerosis, *Science*, 193, 1094, 1976.
5. Brown, M. S. and Goldstein, J. L., Lipid metabolism in the macrophage, *Ann. Rev. Biochem.*, 52, 223, 1983.
6. Harper, A. E., Diet and heart disease — a critical evaluation, in *Dietary Fats and Health*, Perkins, E. G. and Visek, W. J., Eds., American Oil Chemical Society, Champaign, Ill., 1983, 496.
7. Kuller, L. H., Epidemiology of coronary heart disease, in *Dietary Fats and Health*, Perkins, E. G. and Visek, W. J., Eds., American Oil Chemical Society, Champaign, Ill., 1983, 466.
8. Imai, H., Werthessen, N. T., Taylor, C. B., and Lee, K. T., Angiotoxicity and atherosclerosis due to contaminants of USP-grade cholesterol, *Arch. Pathol. Lab. Med.*, 100, 565, 1976.
9. Imai, H., Werthessen, N. T., Subramanyam, V., LeQuesne, P. W., Soloway, A. H., and Kanisawa, M., Angiotoxicity of oxygenated sterols and possible precursors, *Science*, 207, 651, 1980.
10. Peng, S. K. and Taylor, C. B., Atherogenic effect of oxidized cholesterol, in *Dietary Fats and Health*, Perkins, E. G. and Visek, W. J., Eds., American Oil Chemical Society, Champaign, Ill., 1983, 919.
11. Miquel, J., Oro, J., Bensch, K. G., and Johnson, J. E., Jr., Lipofuscin: fine-structure and biochemical studies, in *Free Radicals in Biology*, Pryor, W. A., Ed., Academic Press, New York, 1977, 133.
12. Wilson, R. B., Lipid peroxidation and atherosclerosis, *Crit. Rev. Food Sci.*, 7, 325, 1976.
13. Wilson, R. B., Middleton, C. C., and Sun, G. Y., Vitamin E, antioxidants, and lipid peroxidation in experimental atherosclerosis of rabbits, *J. Nutr.*, 108, 1858, 1978.
14. Hartfort, W. S., Pathogenesis and significance of hemoceroid and hyloceroid, two types of ceroid-like pigment found in human atheromatous lesions, *J. Geriontal.*, 8, 158, 1953.
15. Glavand, J. and Hartmann, S., The occurrence of peroxidized lipids in atheromatous human aortas, *Experentia*, 7, 464, 1951.

16. Woodford, F. P., Bottcher, C. J. F., Oette, K., and Ahiens, E. H., Jr., The artifactual nature of lipid peroxides detected in extracts of human aorta, *J. Atheroscler. Res.*, 5, 31, 1965.
17. Iwakami, M., Peroxides as a factor of atherosclerosis, *Nagoya J. Med. Sci.*, 28, 50, 1965.
18. Brooks, C. J. W., Steel, G., Gilbert, J. D., and Harland, W. A., Lipids of human athroma. IV. Characterization of a new group of polar sterols from human atherosclerotic plaques, *Atherosclerosis*, 13, 223, 1971.
19. Harland, W. A., Gilbert, J. D., Steel, G., and Brooks, C. J. W., Lipids of human atheroma. V. The occurrence of a new group of polar sterol esters from human atherosclerotic plaques, *Atherosclerosis*, 13, 239, 1971.
20. Heinle, H. and Liebich, H., The influence of diet-induced hypercholesterolemia on the degree of oxidation of glutathione in rabbit aorta, *Atherosclerosis*, 37, 637, 1980.
21. Hoff, H. F., Bradley, W. A., Heideman, C. L., Gaubaty, J. W., Karagas, M. D., and Gotto, A. M., Jr., Characterization of low density lipoprotein-like particle in the human aorta from grossly normal and atherosclerotic regions, *Biochim. Biophys. Acta*, 573, 361, 1979.
22. Hollander, W., Paddock, J., and Colombo, M., Lipoproteins in human atherosclerotic vessels. I. Biochemical properties of arterial low density lipoproteins, very low density lipoproteins, and high density lipoproteins, *Exp. Mol. Pathol.*, 30, 144, 1979.
23. Nishigaki, I., Hagihara, M., Tsunekawa, H., Maseki, M., and Yagi, K., Lipid peroxide levels of serum lipoprotein fractions of diabetic patients, *Biochem. Med.*, 25, 373, 1981.
24. Sato, Y., Hotta, N., Sakamoto, N., Matsuoka, S., Ohishi, N., and Yagi, K., Lipid peroxide level in plasma of diabetic patients, *Biochem. Med.*, 21, 104, 1979.
25. Smith, T. L., Toda, T., and Kummerow, F. A., Plasma lipid peroxidation in hyperlipidemic chickens, *Atherosclerosis*, 57, 119, 1985.
26. Dillard, C. J. and Tappel, A. L., Fluorescent products from reaction of peroxidizing polyunsaturated fatty acids with phosphatidylethanolamine and phenylalanine, *Lipids*, 8, 183, 1973.
27. Coolbear, K. P. and Keough, K. M. W., Lipid oxidation and gel to liquid-crystaline transition temperature of synthetic polyunsaturated mixed-acid phosphatidylcholines, *Biochim. Biophys. Acta*, 732, 531, 1983.
28. Bruch, R. C. and Thayer, W. S., Differential effect of lipid peroxidation on membrane fluidity as determined by electron spin resonance probes, *Biochim. Biophys. Acta*, 733, 216, 1983.
29. Curtis, M. T., Gilfor, D., and Farber, J. L., Lipid peroxidation increases the molecular order of microsomal membranes, *Arch. Biochem. Biophys.*, 235, 644, 1984.
30. van Duijn, G., Verkley, A. J., and de Kruijff, B., Influence of phospholipid peroxidation on the phase behavior of phosphatidylcholine and phosphatidylethanolamine in aqueous dispersions, *Biochemistry*, 23, 4969, 1984.
31. Holmes, R. P., Smith, T. L., and Kummerow, F. A., Microheterogeneity in biological membranes, in *Membrane Processes: Molecular Biology and Medical Applications*, Benga, Gh., Baum, H., and Kummerow, F. A., Eds., Springer-Verlag, New York, 1984, 49.
32. Jain, S. K., The accumulation of malonyldialdehyde a product of fatty acid peroxidation, can disturb aminophospholipid organization in the membrane bilayer of human erythrocytes, *J. Biol. Chem.*, 259, 3391, 1984.
33. Barsukov, L. I., Victorov, A. V., Vasilenko, I. A., Evstigneeva, R. P., and Bergelson, L. D., Investigation of the inside-outside distribution, intermembrane exchange and transbilayer movement of phospholipids in sonicated vesicles by shift reagent NMR, *Biochim. Biophys. Acta*, 598, 153, 1980.
34. Shaw, J. M. and Thompson, T. E., Effect of phospholipid oxidation products on transbilayer movement of phospholipids in single lamellar vesicles, *Biochemistry*, 21, 920, 1982.
35. Sandermann, H., Jr., Lipid solvation and kinetic cooperativity of functional membrane proteins, *Trends Biochem. Sci.*, 8, 408, 1983.
36. Isaacson, Y. A., Deroo, P. W., Rosenthal, A. F., Bittman, R., McIntyre, J. O., Bock, H-G., Gazzotti, P., and Fleischer, S., The structural specificity of lecithin of activation of purified D-β-hydroxylbutyrate apodehydrogenase, *J. Biol. Chem.*, 254, 117, 1979.
37. Churchill, P., McIntyre, J. O., Eibl, H., and Fleischer, S., Activation of D-β-hydroxybutyrate apodehydrogenase using molecular species of mixed fatty acyl phospholipids, *J. Biol. Chem.*, 258, 208, 1983.
38. Madden, T. D., Hope, M. J., and Cullis, P. R., Lipid requirements for coupled cytochrome oxidase vesicles, *Biochemistry*, 22, 1970, 1983.
39. Kornburst, D. J. and Mavis, R. D., Microsomal lipid peroxidation. II. Stimulation by carbon tetrachloride, *Mol. Pharmacol.*, 17, 408, 1980.
40. Chiarpotto, E., Poli, G., Albano, E., Gravela, E., and Dianzani, M. U., Studies on fatty liver with isolated hepatocytes. III. Cumene hydroperoxide-induced change of several cell functions, *Exp. Mol. Pathol.*, 41, 191, 1984.

41. Willis, E. D., Effects of lipid peroxidation on membrane-bound enzymes of the endoplasmic reticulum, *Biochem. J.,* 123, 983, 1971.
42. Narabayashi, H., Takeshigl, K., and Minakami, S., Alteration of inner-membrane components and damage to electron-transfer activities of bovine heart submitochondrial particles induced by NAD pH-dependent lipid peroxidation, *Biochem. J.,* 202, 97, 1982.
43. Brogan, W. C., Miles, R. R., and Colby, H. D., Effects of lipid peroxidation on adrenal microsomal monoxygenase, *Biochim. Biophys. Acta,* 753, 114, 1983.
44. Lowrey, K., Glende, E. A., Jr., and Rechnael, R. O., Complete destruction of liver microsomal calcium pump activity by minimal lipid peroxidation in vitro, *Fed. Proc. Fed. Am. Soc. Exp. Biol.,* 39(Abstr. 2284), 1, 1980.
45. Moore, L., Effect of *t*-butyl hydroperoxide on liver microsomal membranes and microsomal calcium sequestration, *Biochim. Biophys. Acta,* 777, 216, 1984.
46. Koster, J. F. and Slee, R. G., Lipid peroxidation of human erythrocyte ghosts induced by organic hydroperoxides, *Biochim. Biophys. Acta,* 752, 233, 1983.
47. Koster, J. F., Slee, R. G., Rutten-Van Beysterweld, C. C. M., and Montfoort, A., The effect of (13 OO H) linoleic acid on human erythrocytes and on erythrocyte ghosts, *Biochim. Biophys. Acta,* 754, 238, 1984.
48. Sullivan, S. G. and Stern, A., Membrane protein changes induced by test-butyl hydroperoxide in red blood cells, *Biochim. Biophys. Acta,* 774, 215, 1984.
49. Hicks, M. and Gebicki, J. M., A quantitative relationship between permeability and the degree of peroxidation in ufasome membranes, *Biochem. Biophys. Res. Commun.,* 80, 704, 1978.
50. Kostava, V. T., Sharyshev, A. A., Rakhmaninova, A. B., Votyakova, T. V., Yevtodiyenko, Yu. A., and Yaguzhinskii, L. S., Induction of ionic transport related to oxidative reactions in the membranes of the mitochondria and liposomes, *Biofizika,* 24, 230, 1979.
51. Marshansky, V. N., Novgorodov, S. A., and Yaguzhinsky, L. S., The role of lipid peroxidation in the induction of cation transport in liver mitochondria, *FEBS Lett.,* 158, 27, 1983.
52. Goldstein, I. M. and Weissmann, G., Effect of the generation of superoxide anion on permeability of liposomes, *Biochem. Biophys. Res. Commun.,* 75, 604, 1977.
53. Shubin, M. V., Paglazov, A. F., Skotselyas, Yu. G., and Vladimirov, Yu. A., Study of the effect of the peroxide oxidation of lipids on the permeability of membranes of the liposomes for Ca^{++} ions, *Biofizika,* 20, 161, 1975.
54. Holmes, R. P. and Yoss, N. L., 25-hydroxysterols increase the permeability of liposomes to Ca^{2+} and other cations, *Biochim. Biophys. Acta,* 770, 15, 1984.
55. Shimshick, E. J. and McConnell, H. M., Lateral phase separation in phospholipid membranes, *Biochemistry,* 12, 2351, 1973.
56. Sokolov, V. S., Churakova, T. D., Bulgakov, V. G., Kagan, V. Ye., Bilenko, M. V., and Boguslavskii, L. I., Study of the mechanisms of action of the products of peroxide oxidation of lipids on the permeability of bilayer lipid membranes, *Biofizika,* 26, 147, 1981.
57. Merrson, F. Z., Kagan, V. E., Kozlov, Yu. P., Belkina, L. M., and Arkhipenko, Yu. V., The role of lipid peroxidation in pathogenesis of ischemic damage and the antioxidant protection of the heart, *Basic Res. Cardiol.,* 77, 465, 1982.
58. Kunimoto, M., Inoue, K., and Nojima, S., Effect of ferrous ion and ascorbate-induced lipid peroxidation on liposomal membranes, *Biochim. Biophys. Acta,* 646, 169, 1981.
59. Smolen, J. E. and Shohet, S. B., Permeability changes induced by peroxidation in liposomes prepared from human erythrocyte lipids, *J. Lipid Res.,* 15, 273, 1974.
60. Gerrity, R. G., Richardson, M., Somer, J. B., Bell, F. P., and Schwartz, C. J., Endothelial cell morphology in areas of *in vivo* evans blue uptake in the aorta of young pigs, *Am. J. Pathol.,* 89, 313, 1977.
61. Mason, R. G. and Balis, J. U., Pathology of the endothelium, *Pathobiol. Cell Membr.,* 2, 425, 1980.
62. Ross, R., Bowen-Pope, D., Raines, E. W., and Faggiotto, A., Endothelial injury: blood-vessel wall interactions, *Proc. N.Y. Acad. Sci.,* 401, 260, 1982.
63. Goode, T. B., Davies, P. F., Reidy, M. A., and Bowyer, D. E., Aortic endothelial cell morphology observed in situ by scanning electron microscopy during atherogenesis in the rabbit, *Atherosclerosis,* 27, 235, 1977.
64. Smith, E. B. and Staples, E. M., Distribution of plasma protein across the human aortic wall, *Atherosclerosis,* 37, 579, 1983.
65. Smith, E. B. and Ashall, C., Low-density lipoprotein concentration in interstitial fluid from human atherosclerotic lesions, *Biochim. Biophys. Acta,* 754, 249, 1983.
66. Hollis, T. M., Enea, N. A., and Kern, J. A., Time-dependent changes in aortic permeability characteristics in experimental diabetes, *Exp. Mol. Pathol.,* 41, 207, 1984.
67. Hennig, B., Shasby, D. M., Fulton, A. B., and Spector, A. A., Exposure to free fatty acid increases the transfer of albumin across cultured endothelial monolayers, *Atherosclerosis,* 4, 489, 1984.

68. Yagi, K., Ohkawa, H., Ohishi, N., Yamashita, M., and Nakashima, T., Lesion of aortic intima caused by intravenous administration of linoleic acid hydroperoxide, *J. Appl. Biochem.*, 3, 58, 1981.
69. Kontos, H. A., Wei, E. P., Povlishock, J. T., Dietrich, W. D., Magier, C. J., and Ellis, E. F., Cerebral arteriolar damage by arachidonic acid and prostaglandin G_2, *Science*, 209, 1242, 1980.
70. Ager, A. and Gordon, J. L., Differential effects of hydrogen peroxide on indices of endothelial cell function, *J. Exp. Med.*, 159, 592, 1984.
71. Gryglewski, R. J., Prostaglandins, platelets, and atherosclerosis, *Crit. Rev. Biochem.*, 7, 291, 1980.
72. Jorgensen, K. A. and Dyerberg, J., Platelets and atherosclerosis, *Adv. Nutr. Res.*, 5, 57, 1983.
73. Best, L. C., Jones, P. B. B., McGuire, M. B., and Russell, R. G. G., Thromboxane B_2 production and lipid peroxidation in human blood platelets, *Adv. Prostagl. Thrombox. Res.*, 6, 297, 1980.
74. Curwen, K. D., Gimbrone, M. A. G., Jr., Hardin, R. I., In vitro studies of thromboresistance, the role of prostacyclin (PGI_2) in platelet adhesion to cultured normal and virally transformed human vascular endothelial cells, *Lab. Invest.*, 42, 366, 1980.
75. Weiss, S. J., Young, J., Lo Buglio, A. F., Slivka, A., and Nimch, N. F., Role of hydrogen peroxide in neutrophil-mediated destruction of cultured endothelial cells, *J. Clin. Invest.*, 68, 713, 1981.
76. Martin, W. J., II, Neutrophils kill pulmonary endothelial cells by a hydrogen-peroxide-dependent pathway, *Am. Res. Respir. Dis.*, 130(2), 209, 1984.
77. Harlan, J. M., Killen, P. D., Harker, L. A., and Striker, G. E., Neutrophil-mediated endothelial injury in vitro, *J. Clin. Invest.*, 68, 1394, 1981.
78. Szczeklik, A. and Gryglewski, R. J., Low density lipoproteins (LDL) are carriers for lipid peroxides and inhibit prostacyclin (PGI_2) biosynthesis in arteries, *Artery*, 7, 488, 1980.
79. Fogelman, A. M., Shechter, I., Seager, J., Hokom, M., Child, J. S., and Edwards, P. A., Malondi-aldehyde alteration of low density lipoprotein leads to cholesterol ester accumulation in human mon-ocyte-macrophages, *Proc. Natl. Acad. Sci.*, 77, 2214, 1980.
80. Haberland, M. E., Fogelman, A. M., and Edwards, P. A., Specificity of receptor-mediated recogni-tion of malonyldialdehyde modified low density lipoprotein, *Proc. Natl. Acad. Sci.*, 79, 1712, 1982.
81. Bon, G. B., Cazzolato, G., and Avogaro, P., Changes of apolipoprotein B molecular weight and immunoreactivity in malondialdehyde-modified low density lipoproteins, *Artery*, 12, 74, 1983.
82. Stein, O. and Stein, Y., Bovine aortic endothelial cells display macrophage-like properties towards acetylated ^{125}I-labeled low density lipoprotein, *Biochim. Biophys. Acta*, 620, 631, 1980.
83. Henriksen, T., Evensen, S. A., and Carlander, B., Injury to cultured endothelial cells induced by low density lipoproteins: protection by high density lipoproteins, *Scand. J. Clin. Lab. Invest.*, 39, 369, 1979.
84. Morel, D. W., Hessler, J. R., and Chisolm, G. M., Low density lipoprotein cytotoxicity induced by free radical peroxidation of lipid, *J. Lipid Res.*, 24, 1070, 1983.
85. Hessler, J. R., Morel, D. W., Lewis, L. J., and Chisolur, G. M., Lipoprotein oxidation and lipopro-tein-induced cytotoxicity, *Atherosclerosis*, 3, 215, 1983.
86. Peng, S. K., Taylor, C. B., Mosbach, E. H., Huang, W. Y., Hill, J., and Mikkelson, B., Distribution of 25-hydroxycholesterol in plasma lipoproteins and its role in atherogenesis, *Atherosclerosis*, 41, 395, 1982.
87. Hessler, J. R., Robertson, A. L., Jr., and Chisolm, G. M., III, LDL-induced cytotoxicity and its inhibition by HDL in human vascular smooth muscle and endothelial cells in culture, *Atherosclerosis*, 32, 213, 1979.
88. Miller, N. E., Weinstein, D. B., Carew, T. E., Koschinsky, T., and Steinberg, D., Interaction be-tween high density and low density lipoproteins during uptake and degradation by cultured fibro-blasts, *J. Clin. Invest.*, 60, 78, 1977.
89. Yoshida, Y., Fischer-Dzoga, K., and Wissler, R. W., Effects of normolipidemic high-density lipopro-teins on proliferation of monkey aortic smooth muscle cells induced by hyperlipidemic low-density lipoproteins, *Exp. Mol. Pathol.*, 41, 258, 1984.
90. Aqel, N. M., Ball, R. Y., Waldmann, H., and Mitchinson, M. J., Monocytic origin of foam cells in human atherosclerotic plaques, *Atherosclerosis*, 53, 265, 1984.
91. Brown, M. S., Basu, S. K., Falck, J. R., Ho, Y. K., and Goldstein, J. L., The scavenger cell pathway for lipoprotein degradation: specificity of the binding site that mediates the uptake of negatively-charged LDL by macrophages, *J. Supramol. Struct.*, 13, 67, 1980.
92. Brown, M. S., Ho, Y. K., and Goldstein, J. L., The cholesterol ester cycle in macrophage foam cells, *J. Biol. Chem.*, 255, 9344, 1980.
93. Goldstein, J. L., Ho, Y. K., Basu, S. K., and Brown, M. S., Binding site on macrophages that mediates uptake and degradation of actylated low density lipoprotein, producing massive cholesterol deposition, *Proc. Natl. Acad. Sci.*, 76, 333, 1979.
94. Mahley, R. W., Innerarity, T. L., Weisgraber, K. H., and Ho, S. Y., Altered metabolism of plasma lipoproteins after selected chemical modification of lysine residues of the apoproteins, *J. Clin. In-vest.*, 64, 743, 1979.

95. Goldstein, J. L., Ho, Y. K., Brown, M. S., Innerarity, T. L., and Mahley, R. W., Cholesterol ester accumulation in macrophages resulting from receptor-mediated uptake and degradation of hypercholesterolemic caine very low density lipoprotein, *J. Biol. Chem.*, 255, 1839, 1980.

96. Fless, G. M., Kirchhausen, T., Fischer-Dzoga, K., Wissler, R. W., and Scanu, A. M., Serum low density lipoproteins with mitogenic effect on cultured aortic smooth muscle cells, *Atherosclerosis*, 41, 171, 1982.

97. Rasmussen, H., *Calcium and cAMP as Synarchic Messengers*, John Wiley and Sons, New York, 1981.

98. Taylor, D. L., Blinks, J. R., and Reynold, G., Contractile basis of ameboid movement. VIII. Aequorin luminescence during ameboid movement, endocytosis, and capping, *J. Cell Biol.*, 86, 599, 1980.

99. Spearman, T. N. and Butcher, F. R., Calcium and exocytosis-the rat parotid as a model, in *The Role of Calcium in Biological Systems*, Vol. 2, Anghileri, L. J. and Tuffet-Anghileu, A. M., Eds., CRC Press, Boca Raton, Fla., 1982, 121.

100. Jain, S. K. and Shohet, S. B., Calcium potentiates the peroxidation of erythrocyte membrane lipids, *Biochim. Biophys. Acta*, 642, 46, 1981.

101. Jackson, M. J., Jones, D. A., and Harris, E. J., Inhibition of lipid peroxidation in muscle homogenates by phospholipase A_2 inhibitors, *Biosci. Rep.*, 4, 581, 1984.

102. Schanne, F. A. X., Kane, A. B., Young, E. E., and Farber, J. L., Calcium dependence of toxic cell death: a final common pathway, *Science*, 206, 700, 1979.

103. Baum, H. and Booth, R. F. G., Transmembrane calcium fluxes, and cell death, in *Membrane Processes, Molecular Biology, and Medical Applications*, Benga, Gh., Baum, H., and Kummerow, F. A., Eds., Springer-Verlag, New York, 1984, 167.

104. Best, L. C., Jones, P. B. B., McGuire, M. B., and Russell, R. G. G., Thromboxane B_2 production and lipid peroxidation in human blood platelets, in *Advances in Prostaglandin and Thromboxane Research*, Vol. 6, Samuelsoon, B., Ramwell, P. W., and Paoletti, R., Eds., Raven Press, New York, 1980, 297.

105. Hayaishi, O. and Shimizu, T., Metabolic and functional significance of prostaglandins in lipid peroxide research, in *Lipid Peroxides in Biology in Medicine*, Yagi, K., Ed., Academic Press, New York, 1982, 41.

106. Lands, W. E. M., Kulmacy, R. J., and Marshall, P. J., Lipid peroxide actions in the regulation of prostaglandin biosynthesis, in *Free Radicals in Biology*, Vol. 4, Pryor, W., Ed., Academic Press, New York, 1984, 39.

107. Henriksen, T., Mahoney, E. M., and Steinberg, D., Interactions of plasma lipoproteins with endothelial cells, *Ann. N.Y. Acad. Sci.*, 401, 102, 1982.

108. Morel, D. W., DiCorleto, P. E., and Chisolm, G. M., Endothelial and smooth muscle cells after low density lipoprotein in vitro by free radical oxidation, *Arteriosclerosis*, 4, 357, 1984.

109. Winser, D. A., Jr., Shirai, K., and Jackson, R. L., Purification and properties of bovine aortic lipoprotein lipase, *Artery*, 6, 419, 1980.

110. Scow, R. O., Blanchette-Mackie, E. J., and Smith, L. C., Transport of lipid across capillary endothelium, *Fed. Proc. Fed. Am. Soc. Exp. Biol.*, 39, 2610, 1980.

111. Zilversmit, D. B., A proposal linking atherogenesis to the interaction of endothelial lipoprotein lipase with triglyceride-rich lipoproteins, *Circ. Res.*, 6, 633, 1973.

112. Morisaki, N., Lindsey, J. A., Stitto, J. M., and Cornwell, D. G., Fatty acid metabolism and cell proliferation. V. Evaluation of pathways for the generation of lipid peroxides, *Lipids*, 19, 381, 1984.

113. Novikoff, A. B., Novikoff, P. M., Quintana, N., and Davis, C., Studies on microperoxisomes. IV. Interrelations of microperoxisomes, endoplasmic reticulum, and lipofuscin granules, *J. Histochem. Cytochem.*, 21, 1010, 1973.

114. Reddy, J. K., Lalwani, N. D., Reddy, M. K., and Qureshi, S. A., Excessive accumulation of autofluorescent lipofuscin in the liver during hepatocarcinogenesis by methylchlofenapate and other hypolipidemia peroxisomal proliferators, *Cancer Res.*, 42, 259, 1982.

115. Levin, W., Lu, A. Y. H., Jacobson, M., Kuntzman, R., Poyer, J. L., and McCay, P. B., Lipid peroxidation and the degradation of cytochrome P-450 heme, *Arch. Biochem. Biophys.*, 158, 842, 1973.

116. Camacho, J. and Rubalcava, B., Lipid composition of liver plasma membranes from rats intoxicated with carbon tetrachloride, *Biochim. Biophys. Acta*, 776, 97, 1984.

117. Benedetti, A., Casini, A. F., Fevali, M., and Comporti, M., Effects of diffusible products of peroxidation of rat liver microsomal lipids, *Biochem. J.*, 180, 303, 1979.

118. Suematsu, T., Kamada, T., Abe, H., Kibuchi, S., and Yagi, K., Serum lipid peroxide level in patients suffering from liver diseases, *Clin. Chim. Acta*, 79, 267, 1977.

119. Babior, B. M., Oxygen-dependent microbial killing by phagocytes, *N. Engl. J. Med.*, 298, 659, 1978.

120. McCord, J. M. and Fridovich, I., The reduction of cytochrome c by milk xanthine oxidase, *J. Biol. Chem.,* 243, 5753, 1968.
121. Tien, M. and Aust, S. D., Comparative aspects of several model lipid peroxidation systems, in *Lipid Peroxides in Biology and Medicine,* Yagi, K., Ed., Academic Press, New York, 1982, 23.
122. Perkins, E. G. and Kummerow, F. A., The isolation and characterization of the polymers formed during the thermal oxidation of corn oil, *J. Am. Oil Chem. Soc.,* 36, 371, 1958.
123. Alexander, J. C., Chemical and biological properties related to toxicity of heated fats, *J. Toxic Environ. Health,* 7, 125, 1981.
124. Izaki, Y., Yoshikawa, S., and Uchiyama, M., Effect of ingestion of thermally oxidized frying oil on peroxidative criteria in rats, *Lipids,* 19, 324, 1984.
125. Chiu, O., Lubin, B., and Shohet, S. B., Peroxidative reactions in red cell biology, in *Free Radicals in Biology,* Vol. 5, Pryor, W. A., Ed., Academic Press, New York, 1982, 115.
126. Stary, H. C. and Letson, G. D., Morphometry of coronary, artery components in children and young adults, *Arteriosclerosis,* 8, 485a, 1983.
127. Strong, J. P., Restrepo, C., and Guyman, M., Coronary and aortic atherosclerosis in New Orleans. II. Comparison of lesions by age, sex, and race, *Lab. Invest.,* 39, 364, 1978.
128. McGill, H. C., Jr., Persistent problems in the pathogenesis of atherosclerosis, *Atherosclerosis,* 4, 443, 1984.
129. Connor, S. S., Connor, W. E., Saxton, G., Calvin, L., and Bacon, S., The effects of age, body weight and family relationships on plasma lipoproteins in men, women and children of randomly selected families, *Circulation,* 65, 1290, 1982.
130. Yagi, K., Assay for serum lipid peroxide level and its clinical significance, in *Lipid Peroxides in Biology and Medicine,* Yagi, K., Ed., Academic Press, New York, 1982, 223.
131. Smith, T., unpublished data.
132. Smith, T. and Moriarity, unpublished data.

Chapter 6

DIETARY CONTROL OF LIPOPROTEINS

Robert J. Nicolosi and Jerome L. Hojnacki

TABLE OF CONTENTS

I. GENERAL REVIEW

A. Introduction

Data from both human and animal studies have established that certain dietary factors can dramatically affect plasma lipoprotein levels and metabolism. An association between abnormal plasma lipoprotein levels and increased risk of coronary heart disease has also been supported by both epidemiological and experimental evidence.[1-4]

Our objective is to give an overview of those dietary factors which influence plasma lipoprotein levels and metabolism. The dietary factors to be discussed will include dietary fat saturation and cholesterol, fish oil, carbohydrate, protein, fiber, and alcohol. Before discussing these dietary variables lipoprotein character and metabolism will be outlined briefly.

II. OUTLINE OF LIPOPROTEIN METABOLISM

Plasma lipoproteins are mainly spherical macromolecular complexes which consist of surface components of phospholipid, free cholesterol, and protein and a core containing mostly triglyceride and cholesteryl ester. Lipoproteins are synthesized mainly by the liver and intestine and catabolized by both hepatic and extrahepatic tissues. Their main function is to transport dietary and/or synthesized triglyceride, phospholipids, and cholesterol from one organ to the next where they may be used as sources of energy, membrane structure and function, and hormone synthesis.

Historically, normal plasma lipoproteins have been classified into four major families based on density, composition, and electrophoretic mobility: (1) chylomicrons, (2) very low density lipoproteins (VLDL), (3) low density lipoproteins (LDL), and (4) high density lipoproteins (HDL). Low density lipoprotein fractions have been further divided into intermediate density lipoprotein (IDL or LDL_1) (density 1.006 to 1.019 g/mℓ) and LDL_2 (density 1.019 to 1.063 g/mℓ). The LDL_2 is the major component of plasma LDL. HDL has also been subfractionated into HDL_2 (density 1.063 to 1.120 g/mℓ) and HDL_3 (density 1.120 to 1.210 g/mℓ). The protein components of lipoproteins are referred to as apoproteins and have been designated apo A-I, apo A-II, apo A-IV, apo B, apo CI, apo C-II and apo C-III, apo D, and apo E.

A. Lipoprotein Metabolism

1. Chylomicrons

After hydrolysis of dietary lipid in the small intestine, the major breakdown products are absorbed into the intestinal cells (enterocytes) and the lipids re-esterified in the endoplasmic reticulum for subsequent packaging into chylomicrons with apoproteins, A-I, A-IV, and the intestinal apo B, B-48. Chylomicrons are secreted from the enterocyte into the lacteals of the intestinal villi and subsequently enter the venous circulation via the thoracic duct. The triglyceride that enters the plasma in chylomicrons can be utilized for energy or transported to adipose tissue and muscle for storage and utilization. Shortly after entering the plasma, these lipoproteins acquire apo E and apo C-II from a reservoir of circulating HDL. During this process, chylomicrons are catabolized to form chylomicron remnants by lipoprotein lipase, an enzyme located on the outer surfaces of endothelial cells of peripheral tissue. Apolipoprotein CII which acts as a cofactor stimulates lipoprotein lipase activity which results in hydrolysis of triglycerides to free fatty acids that are rapidly taken up by tissue at the site of hydrolysis. In addition, other chylomicron components (phospholipids, apo A-I, A-II, A-IV, and the C apolipoproteins) are removed and contribute to the formation of disc-like nascent HDL, whereas certain HDL constituents (apo E and cholesteryl-ester) are transferred to chylomicrons. The remaining cholesteryl ester-rich chylomicron remnant containing apo B-48 and apo E can then be taken up by the apo B/E and apo E receptors on the surface of hepatic parenchymal cells for subsequent metabolism.

2. VLDL

Input of triglyceride-rich lipoproteins also occurs from endogenous sources. During and after meals, circulating free fatty acids enter the liver where they may be esterified with glycerol to form triglyceride. Triglyceride synthesized in the liver, together with cholesteryl ester is combined with a lipoprotein monolayer composed of phospholipid, unesterified cholesterol, a form of apo B called B-100, apo E, and apo C, and secreted into the hepatic venous blood as endogenous triglyceride-rich VLDL. As with chylomicrons, circulating VLDL triglycerides and phospholipids with the necessary apo C-II cofactor are hydrolyzed by lipoprotein lipase and surface components such as free cholesterol and phospholipid as well as the apo Cs and apo E are transferred to HDL. The resultant cholesteryl ester-rich apo B-100 containing particle is called an intermediate density lipoprotein (IDL) which following further modification possibly by an enzyme hepatic lipase is converted to LDL.

3. LDL

It appears that with the exception of patients with homozygous familial hypercholesterolemia in which some LDL is directly synthesized, LDL normally arises from the catabolism of VLDL. LDL appears to contain the same amount of apo B, i.e., B-100 per lipoprotein particle as does VLDL, although other apoproteins originally associated with circulating VLDL have almost been entirely removed, together with much of the phospholipid and some cholesterol. LDL appears to be catabolized in varous cell types by both receptor- and nonreceptor-mediated pathways where it can function as the chief source of cholesterol for membrane and hormone synthesis. After LDL apo B-100 is recognized by and bound to specific receptors, LDL is internalized, the apoprotein moiety degraded and the cholesteryl ester hydrolyzed to free cholesterol. This intracellular free cholesterol reduces endogenous cholesterol production by inhibiting the activity of the rate limiting enzyme in intracellular cholesterol synthesis, 3-hydroxy-3 methylglutaryl coenzyme A reductase.

4. HDL

High density lipoproteins synthesized by both the liver and the intestine are disc-shaped and are composed chiefly of surface components of phospholipid and apoproteins A and E. These particles, as already pointed out, can also be derived during catabolism of triglyceride-rich lipoproteins, chylomicrons, and VLDL. The HDL particle is associated with the lecithin:cholesterol acyltransferase enzyme (LCAT) which converts free cholesterol to cholesteryl esters. These cholesteryl esters can then be either catabolized by various tissues or transferred as cholesteryl esters from HDL to VLDL and LDL by a transfer protein for subsequent removal from circulation by various tissues. Those cholesteryl esters incorporated by the liver can be excreted into the bile as either free cholesterol, bile acids, or neutral steroids, a cycle of events that explains the role of HDL in the reverse transport of cholesterol from peripheral tissue to liver.

III. DIETARY FAT AND CHOLESTEROL

A. LDL Cholesterol and Apo B

Many studies of the effect of dietary fat and/or cholesterol on human plasma lipids and lipoprotein levels generally demonstrate that feeding saturated fat and cholesterol elevate and polyunsaturated fat reduce plasma and LDL cholesterol levels.[5-7] Population studies involving Japanese[8] and Polynesian groups[9] have found correlations between serum cholesterol and the levels of saturated fat intake. On the other hand, while the Western Electric Study[10] showed a correlation between the ratio of polyunsaturated to saturated fat intake, plasma lipids, and the incidence of CHD, the Tecumseh Study[11] was unable to demonstrate such an association. Despite these inconsistencies, epidemiological evidence, in general, support the notion that low saturated fat, low cholesterol diets correlate with reduced plasma lipoprotein lipids and incidence of CHD.

While there is general agreement that dietary fat saturation and cholesterol can significantly alter the composition and concentration of lipoprotein lipid, there is no unanimity on the effects of dietary fat on lipoprotein apoproteins. For example, in the case of LDL protein or apo B, Spritz and Mishkel,[12] reported that a 26% fall in LDL cholesterol was attended by only a 9% fall in LDL protein. Shepherd and co-workers[13] also found that polyunsaturated fat diets reduced the cholesterol:protein ratio in LDL. In contrast, Brussard et al.[14] found no fall in the LDL cholesterol:apo B ratio when diets rich in polyunsaturated fat were consumed. These discordant results are not easily explained and have been discussed in detail by Vega and co-workers.[15] Nonhuman primates have been used extensively for studies of dietary saturated fat and/or cholesterol induced elevations of plasma lipoproteins[16-23] and in general support the notion that while the degree of plasma lipoprotein response varies as a function of species, the resultant hypercholesterolemia is nearly always accompanied by an elevation of LDL cholesterol.

While most of these investigations indicate that the plasma cholesterol response is dependent on the interaction between the type of fat and the level of cholesterol, there are some studies that suggest that dietary cholesterol may be an independent variable. For example, the studies of Schonfeld et al.[24] demonstrated that at P:S ratios of 0.25 to 0.40, addition of 750 mg of cholesterol to the diet caused significant increases in plasma and LDL cholesterol levels. However when the P:S ratio was raised to 0.8, the addition of 1500 mg of cholesterol to the diet was required to significantly raise plasma and LDL cholesterol. On the other hand, other studies[25] have shown that the addition of cholesterol to highly saturated fat-containing diets did not significantly increase plasma cholesterol levels over saturated fat feeding alone.

While the lower LDL apo B levels during polyunsaturated fat feeding in humans appears attributable to lower production rates rather than to enhanced catabolism,[26,27] the latter mechanism has been demonstrated in at least one report in nonhuman primates fed a polyunsaturated fat diet.[23]

B. HDL Cholesterol and Apo A-I

While the association of dietary fat saturation and cholesterol feeding with LDL levels is strong, the reported effects of diet on HDL are quite inconsistent. For example, diets high in polyunsaturates and low in cholesterol have been reported to increase,[14] to have no effect,[28] or to decrease HDL cholesterol levels.[29] Feeding diets with P/S ratios of 1.7,[30] 2.0,[31] and 4.0[32] have been reported to decrease HDL levels to varying degrees while a P:S ratio of 1.0 has been found to cause no change[33] or an increase in HDL cholesterol.[34] Most workers have found lower plasma apo A-I levels when diets rich in polyunsaturated fats are consumed.[35-37] Lower apo A-I:A-II ratios on polyunsaturated fat-rich diets have suggested a selective fall in the HDL$_2$[16] and a 28% fall in the HDL$_2$:HDL$_3$ ratio has been reported when polyunsaturates are substituted for saturates in the diet.[38] However, others find no changes in the HDL subclasses.[33] Thus, the variation in reported response may well be explained by the level of polyunsaturated fat fed or the P:S ratio. The possible significance of the duration of diet treatment is suggested by the reports that ingestion of a high polyunsaturated fat diet for 2 weeks, 2 months, or 4 years, decreased,[39] resulted in no change,[40] or increased HDL levels,[41] respectively. The evidence that duration of dietary treatment is an important consideration also comes from the studies of vegetarians which revealed low levels of HDL cholesterol and in particular, HDL_2, and apoA-I:apoA-II ratios.[42] Despite the reductions in HDL cholesterol and apoprotein levels, the reduced risk of CHD in vegetarians may be attributed to the lower levels of LDL cholesterol relative to HDL.

HDL cholesterol response to the feeding of cholesterol has also been reported to be quite variable. Cholesterol feeding reduced HDL cholesterol in the rat,[43] but produced no significant change in swine[44] and dogs.[45] In the nonhuman primate species, cholesterol and/or saturated fat feeding reduced HDL cholesterol in rhesus,[46-48] cynomolgus,[49] and pig-tailed monkeys;[50] produced no significant change in chimpanzees[51] and increased plasma HDL in squirrel[18] and vervet monkeys.[52] The lack of agreement no doubt reflects inherent differences in the responsiveness of the species, the amount of cholesterol fed, and other differences in the dietary regimens, such as the amount and kind of fat or other dietary components which affect serum lipid levels. In many of the studies with monkeys in which HDL levels were reported to decrease, excessive amounts of cholesterol were fed resulting in plasma cholesterol levels of 800 to 1000 mg/dℓ.

The mechanism(s) accounting for the lower HDL levels during polyunsaturated fat feeding is unclear. Shepherd et al.[38] found no change in the fractional catabolic rate (FCR) of ^{125}I-apo A-I reconstituted with homologous HDL and concluded that the lower apo A-I levels were due to a 26% reduction in the apo A-I synthetic rate. However, studies in monkeys by Parks and Rudel[37] suggested higher HDL apoprotein catabolic rates in polyunsaturated fat-fed animals. This question warrants additional investigation since very different techniques were employed in these discordant studies.

C. Other Lipoprotein Responses to Dietary Fat/Cholesterol Treatment

In response to high-fat, high-cholesterol containing diets, human and animal studies[53-64] have demonstrated the production of abnormal lipoproteins, i.e., HDL_c and B-VLDL. In response to these diets, one of the HDL subclasses, HDL_1, accumulates large amounts of cholesterol and an arginine-rich apoprotein, apo E and is designated HDL_c. This lipoprotein class is thought to be involved in the mechanism by which large amounts of peripheral tissue cholesterol are transported to the liver for metabolism. Cholesterol feeding will also result in the production of B-VLDL particles rich in cholesteryl ester and apo E.[64] These particles are thought to have atherogenic potential by virtue of their ability to cause the accumulation of cholesterol in cultured macrophages by nonreceptor mediated processes. The development of probes for the human apolipoprotein genes have not only permitted a qualitative and quantitative comparison of the amounts of specific apolipoprotein mRNA present in different tissues but have also allowed assessment of the influence of dietary fat saturation and/or cholesterol on these processes. Two preliminary reports[65,66] have demonstrated significant reductions in hepatic apo A-I mRNA levels with polyunsaturated fat feeding.

IV. FISH OIL

Unlike many plant sources which contain substantial amounts of linoleic acid (C18:2) of the omega-6 (N-6) fatty acid series, fish oil contains large concentrations of unique fatty acids of the omega-3 (N-3) family which are not characteristically found in appreciable amounts in plants, land animals, or dairy products.[67-70] Two of the major fatty acids in the N-3 series are eicosapentaenoic acid (C20:5, omega-3) (EPA) and docosahexaenoic acid (C22:6, omega-3) (DHA).[67,69] The omega designation represents the carbon atom of the first double bond appearing in the fatty acid structure counting from the methyl group.

A consistent finding in a number of epidemiological reports involving Greenland Eskimos who consume large amounts of fish products,[71,72] and in experimental animal[73] and human[67,74-76] studies where fish oil was substituted for a portion of dietary fat, has been the remarkable hypotriglyceridemic response of these subjects. Dyerberg, Bang, and their colleagues noted an extremely low incidence of CHD in Eskimos when compared to a reference Danish Caucasian group of men.[71,72] The diet of the former consists of seal, whale, and fish which is high in cholesterol content but lower in saturated fat and enriched in polyunsaturated EPA and DHA.[67,77] By contrast, the typical diet consumed by the U.S. population has linoleic acid as the major polyunsaturated fatty acid component.[67,69]

Besides low levels of circulating triglyceride and VLDL, Greenland Eskimos also characteristically exhibit a lipoprotein pattern consisting of reduced concentrations of plasma cholesterol and LDL and elevations in HDL.[71,78] Thus, omega-3 fatty acids may induce an antiatherogenic lipoprotein profile (LDL < HDL) which on a long-term basis might account for the reduced incidence of CHD in this population.[71,78] Some investigators have argued that these alterations in lipoprotein levels may in turn reflect altered metabolism resulting from extensive incorporation of omega-3 fatty acids into lipoprotein structure.[79] Analysis of the Greenland Eskimo plasma[80] and that of other individuals consuming fish oil products shows a marked increase in EPA and DHA esterified to circulating phospholipid, triglyceride, and cholesteryl ester at the expense of oleic, linoleic, and arachidonic acids.[75,76,81] Moreover, studies with fish-oil-fed rats and mink revealed that omega-3 fatty acids are readily incorporated into the triglyceride and phospholipid moieties of most body tissues, particularly the liver and adipose tissue.[82] However, at least in the plasma, this replacement with omega-3 fatty acids may be transient in nature since 2 weeks after consumption of fish oil concentrate is discontinued, fatty acid profiles return to their original pattern.[75]

Of particular importance has been several investigations which evaluated the use of salmon oil diets or a commercial marine lipid concentrate (MaxEPA) to lower plasma triglycerides in patients with various hyperlipoproteinemias[67] or in healthy volunteers with carbohydrate-induced hypertriglyceridemia.[83] For example, Phillipson et al.[67] recently compared the plasma lipid response of Type IIb and Type V patients to control low fat diets, fish oil regimens, and diets rich in vegetable oil (corn + safflower) containing large amounts of omega-6 linoleic acid. Fish oil produced a more marked decline in plasma cholesterol, triglyceride, and VLDL along with decreases in apoproteins B and C-III compared to the vegetable oil diet in Type IIb patients.[67] However, the fish diet also lowered LDL and HDL in these individuals while the corn-safflower regimen caused no change in LDL and raised HDL.[67] Patients with Type V hyperlipoproteinemia showed a remarkable loss of fasting chylomicronemia and a dramatic decline in plasma triglyceride and VLDL while LDL was actually elevated by 48% after consumption of omega-3 fatty acids.[67] When the dietary fat of this group was then replaced by vegetable oil, plasma cholesterol, triglyceride, and VLDL all rose while LDL decreased by 28%.[67] The authors of this study concluded that a reduction in VLDL is more pronounced in patients with the most elevated plasma triglyceride levels and that while both fish and vegetable oil diets can lower plasma cholesterol, the former also has a dramatic hypotriglyceridemic effect.[67]

These same investigators also demonstrated that the characteristic hypertriglyceridemia which results when normal individuals consume excessive amounts of carbohydrate (75% of calories) can be significantly reduced along with plasma cholesterol when fish oil is concurrently used as a source of dietary fat.[83] Since the carbohydrate-induced hypertriglyceridemia is apparently the result of excessive hepatic VLDL synthesis and secretion, fish oil may act by inhibiting this process when subjects are challenged by high carbohydrate intake.[83]

Other animal experiments and studies using healthy normolipemic volunteers reaffirmed observations by Phillipson et al.[67] that compared on a gram-for-gram basis, fish oil fatty acids are more effective in achieving hypocholesterolemic and hypotriglyceridemic effects than vegetable oils containing omega-6 fatty acids.[79,84,85] Although the exact reason for these differences in hypolipidemic response is not known for sure, the greater degree of unsaturation of fish oil fatty acids may play an important role.[79,84] Moreover, besides reducing plasma lipid levels, marine oils, at least in the hypercholesterolemic rat, can mobilize hepatic cholesterol and may impair intestinal cholesterol absorption.[85]

While these studies consistently demonstrate that fish oils produce a marked lowering of plasma triglyceride, the response of plasma and LDL cholesterol to omega-3 fatty acids is considerably more variable. For example, generally lower values for these lipid parameters have been reported in serum analyses of Greenland Eskimos,[71,72] and in some studies involving human volunteers or animals fed fish products.[73,76,79,84-86] LDL and/or plasma cholesterol are also reduced in maturity onset diabetics[87] and in Type IIb hyperlipoproteinemics fed fish oil or marine lipid concentrates.[67] However, other studies using these dietary regimens have revealed either no change in LDL[75,88] or an elevation in this lipoprotein class particularly in patients with Type V hyperlipoproteinemia[67] or in normolipemic volunteers.[76] Since fish oil is apparently effective in inhibiting hepatic VLDL synthesis,[67] and because LDL is normally derived from the catabolism of the former by lipoprotein lipase, one would not expect an increase in low density lipoproteins during consumption of fish oils.[86] The anomalous rise in LDL under these dietary conditions in some individuals may in part be the result of enhanced direct secretion of LDL particles by the liver.[89] The reason for the absence of a consistent LDL response in many of the other studies may reflect the length of treatment time or dietary dose of omega-3 fatty acids.[75,76,88]

Similarly, HDL changes in response to dietary fish oil have been quite variable, including no effect,[67,75,79,80,86,88] elevations,[71,74,76,90,125,147] and depressions[73,89] in these antiatherogenic macromolecules. For example, N-3 fatty acids given to hypertriglyceridemic Type IIb and Type V patients produced no significant change in the concentration of plasma apoprotein A-I, HDLs major protein component or in HDL cholesterol levels.[67] However, vegetable oil caused a marked increase in HDL cholesterol in these same Type IIb patients.[67] Similarly, Bronsgeest-Schoute et al.,[75] Illingworth et al.,[91] and Harris et al.[79] were unable to detect alterations in HDL cholesterol in healthy adults fed either a fish oil concentrate or salmon oil for a 4-week period.

On the other hand, Bang et al.[71] reported higher HDL levels in male Greenland Eskimos compared to Caucasian Danes although this difference was not apparent in women. Yarnell et al.[90] by contrast, observed a positive correlation between fish consumption and HDL cholesterol in women but no such affect could be demonstrated in men consuming 100 g of fish twice a week for 3 months.[88] More long-term studies of 6 weeks to 2 years using either cod-liver oil fed to healthy volunteers[92] or MaxEPA given to patients with coronary heart disease[92] have resulted in significant increases in HDL. Thus, while the majority of studies have demonstrated a consistent hypocholesterolemic and hypotriglyceridemic effect by N-3 fatty acids, the HDL response to fish oils is more variable and may be time, sex, or dose dependent.[71,74,88,92,93]

The several studies[73,89] showing a fish oil related decrease in HDL are of particular importance since a reduction in these lipoprotein particles in circulation may diminish any antiatherogenic effects provided by N-3 fatty acids. Relative to a vegetable oil diet, fish oil caused a decline in HDL cholesterol in patients with Type IIb hyperlipoproteinemia[67] and a decrease in both HDL cholesterol and apoprotein A-I in mildly hypertriglyceridemic subjects fed a combined high carbohydrate-fish oil concentrate regimen.[83] However, Nestel et al.[89] also noticed a decrease in HDL cholesterol and apoprotein A-I in both hypertriglyceridemic and normal subjects following intake of MaxEPA. Thus, whether the HDL response of patients with elevated triglycerides to N-3 fatty acids differs from that of normolipemic individuals is open to question.

The hypolipidemic action of omega-3 fatty acids has been attributed to a number of different alterations in lipid and lipoprotein metabolism including modifications in: (1) hepatic triglyceride and VLDL synthesis and secretion;[67] (2) lipoprotein clearance from the plasma compartment;[86] (3) fecal sterol excretion;[67,73] (4) hepatic cholesterol mobilization;[85] (5) cholesterol absorption from the gut;[85] and (6) LDL apoprotein B production rate.[91]

Harris et al.[79] have proposed at least three theoretical mechanisms which may underlie most fish-oil related alterations in lipoprotein metabolism. These include: (1) enhanced incorporation of EPA and DHA into lipoproteins which would alter their structure and hence affect their degradation by various lipolytic enzymes; (2) alterations in plasma membrane phospholipids which would change the interaction of circulating lipoproteins with membrane bound enzymes such as lipoprotein lipase; and (3) modifications in adipose tissue lipolysis which would influence rates of hepatic uptake of free fatty acids and hence lipoprotein secretion. A substantial amount of experimental data shows that N-3 fatty acids are actively incorporated into plasma lipoprotein structure and tissue lipids, particularly membrane phospholipids, and hence could thus potentially modify lipoprotein metabolism.[73,75,76,86,94] Moreover, several radioisotope studies have provided conclusive evidence that fish-oil consumption markedly influences lipoprotein synthesis turnover.[81,89]

Perhaps the most consistent finding in a number of these studies is that fish oil may suppress hepatic VLDL synthesis and secretion which may thus account for the hypotriglyceridemic action of N-3 fatty acids.[67,89,91] Indirect evidence for this comes from observations by Harris et al.[83] which showed that fish-oil consumption blocks the rapid increase in plasma triglycerides which accompanies excess carbohydrate intake and which is normally the result of enhanced hepatic VLDL synthesis. Moreover, because N-3 fatty acid consumption in this study reduced precursor VLDL levels without concurrent elevations in product LDL, the most likely explanation for the fish oil effect would be inhibition of VLDL synthesis instead of enhanced VLDL catabolism.[83] Two other kinetic studies provided more direct evidence that marine lipids inhibit VLDL apoprotein B production rate[89,91] and also retard the incorporation of ^{3}H glycerol into VLDL triglyceride.[89] Furthermore, these effects are apparently specific for the liver since *de novo* fatty acid synthesis is inhibited by N-3 fatty acids in isolated hepatocytes[95] and in perfused livers from rats fed fish oils.[96] Perfused livers in the latter study also show reduced incorporation of newly synthesized fatty acids into VLDL, depressed secretion of VLDL triglyceride mass, and increased fatty acid oxidation.[96] Interestingly, when shellfish triglycerides, which contain smaller amounts of EPA and DHA are fed to rats, hepatic lipogenic enzymes are also reduced in activity and quantity, and cholesterol synthesis is diminished.[97]

An alternative explanation for the hypotriglyceridemic action of fish oil is enhanced plasma clearance of VLDL by lipoprotein lipase in peripheral tissue. Although, Phillipson et al.[67] noted a concomitant rise in LDL and a drop in VLDL in patients with Type V hyperlipoproteinemia fed salmon oil or MaxEPA, these investigators were unable to detect any alteration in post-heparin lipoprotein lipase activity relative to control diets. On the other hand, Nestel et al.[89] observed an increase in the fractional removal of ^{125}I-VLDL apoprotein and Harris and Connor[86] reported accelerated plasma clearance of triglyceride-rich lipoproteins in normal subjects fed fish oil. Both studies suggest that fish-oil-induced reduction in circulating triglyceride may also result from enhanced removal of plasma lipoproteins, specifically VLDL. In addition, the marked reduction in chylomicrons in Type V patients fed salmon oil or MaxEPA may also reflect an increased clearance capacity.[67] Putatively, accelerated clearance of both VLDL and chylomicrons may be the result of incorporation of EPA and DHA into membrane phospholipids of peripheral tissue which might enhance lipoprotein lipase activity.[86]

Because biliary excretion of neutral sterol and bile acids represents quantitatively the most important exit route of cholesterol from the body,[98] several investigators have postulated that in addition to reducing circulating cholesterol levels, fish oils may also promote biliary cholesterol efflux.[67,73] Peifer et al.[85] earlier provided evidence that marine oils fed to rats with diet-induced hypercholesterolemia actively mobilize cholesterol from hepatic tissue although fecal sterol output was not measured. Connor et al.,[99] however, performed sterol balance studies with humans which showed that N-3 fatty acids enhance fecal sterol excretion. To date, Balasubramaniam et al.[73] conducted the most comprehensive evaluation of fish oil and sterol efflux. These investigators evaluated the effects of dietary fish, coconut, and safflower oils on rat lipoprotein and tissue composition, and biliary cholesterol excretion. Similar to findings in other studies, EPA and DHA were incorporated into lipoprotein, liver, and biliary lipids. In addition, fish oil caused a markedly greater decrease in plasma cholesterol than the safflower oil regimen which was attributed to a drop in the concentration of both LDL and HDL.[73] Of particular interest, was the discovery in this study that N-3 fatty acids enhanced the basal secretion rate of biliary cholesterol without altering excretion of acidic sterols. The authors[73] speculated that the fish-oil diet apparently accelerates lipoprotein catabolism and facilitates uptake of lipoprotein cholesterol by hepatic tissue apparently because of modifications in hepatocyte membrane phospholipids which become enriched with 20:5 and 22:6 fatty acids.

Alternatively, marine oils might also exert their hypolipidemic effects by interfering with the absorption of dietary cholesterol as discussed by Peifer et al.[85] However, Chen et al.[100] administered ^{14}C oleic, arachidonic, or EPA along with ^{3}H cholesterol to rats and found identical patterns of cholesterol absorption. Moreover, these investigators showed that EPA is efficiently absorbed and incorporated into the triglyceride of lymphatic chylomicrons and VLDL comparable to what was observed for oleic and arachidonic acids. These findings in the rat are in contrast to earlier studies which suggested that N-3 fatty acids may be poorly hydrolyzed by pancreatic lipase and inefficiently absorbed from the intestine.[100,101]

More recent interest has focused on the role of fish oils in altering circulating levels of atherogenic low density lipoproteins. Illingworth et al.[91] were the first to conclusively demonstrate using ^{125}I-LDL and kinetic analyses that consumption of marine oils significantly reduces the absolute catabolic rate (ACR) of LDL, taken as a measure of synthesis in the steady state, without altering LDL clearance (fractional catabolic rate). This differs from N-6 fatty acids which can apparently increase LDL degradation by enhancing LDL receptor activity.[102] Illingworth et al.[91] concluded that the observed decrease in LDL ACR following intake of salmon oil or MaxEPA may be due to a direct inhibition of precursor VLDL synthesis or accelerated clearance of VLDL remnants and hence reduced conversion to product low density lipoproteins. By contrast, Nestel et al.[89] found a more variable effect of fish oil on plasma LDL levels and at least in two subjects they examined, a marked increase in LDL was observed which may have been the result of enhanced independent direct synthesis and secretion of LDL particles.

Finally, virtually nothing is known about the effects of fish oil on HDL metabolism. As noted earlier, increases, decreases, and no changes have been reported in circulating levels of these antiatherogenic molecules in a number of human and animal dietary marine lipid studies.[73,74,86,89,90,92,103,104] To date, only one very recent study by Sanders et al.[104] using hypertriglyceridemic men fed 15 g of MaxEPA per day showed that marine polyunsaturates selectively raise HDL_3 cholesterol and depress the HDL_2:HDL_3 cholesterol ratio which is apparently unrelated to the concurrent observation of a reduced rate of VLDL synthesis.

V. CARBOHYDRATE

Recommendations to reduce caloric intake from fat require an increase in carbohydrates. An increase in dietary carbohydrate causes a rise in the plasma triglyceride level of fasting individuals[105,106] but except for those with abnormal lipid levels, the increase is usually minimal and transient.[107,108] From studies of normal and Type IV subjects fed 40 and 80% of calories as carbohydrate, Quarfordt et al.[109] concluded that the high carbohydrate-induced hypertriglyceridemia was associated with an increased VLDL-triglyceride pool size and net transport. The hypertriglyceridemia in individuals fed diets high in carbohydrate has been associated with both increases in hepatic VLDL secretion[110] and reduced clearance of endogenous VLDL particles.[111] When carbohydrates are substituted for saturated fatty acids, plasma cholesterol and LDL usually fall.[112] In general, reductions in HDL, and in particular the HDL_2 subclass have also been reported.[113-115] The reduction in HDL and apo A-I has been associated with increased HDL catabolism.[116] Striking changes in VLDL composition and the distribution of apo C proteins in normolipemic adults fed a high carbohydrate diet for 4 days have been reported by Schonfeld et al.[114] These studies demonstrated that plasma VLDL triglyceride, cholesterol, and protein rose by factors of 2.4, 1.67, and 1.88, respectively, indicating an enrichment of triglyceride. The observed increase in the amount of apo C-II relative to C-III may have physiological significance since apo C-II activates and C-III inactivates lipoprotein lipase, the enzyme which catabolizes triglyceride-rich lipoproteins resulting in the peripheral storage of triglyceride and formation of remnant particles. The role of apo C apoproteins in lipoprotein clearance is also supported by the observations that apo C-III inhibits apo E-mediated recognition of lipoproteins by cellular receptors.[117] Further subfraction of apo C-III into apo C-III_0, C-III_1, and C-III_2 have revealed that the feeding of high carbohydrate diets is associated with an increase in apo C-III_0[115] and a decrease in the percentage of C-III_2 in VLDL and HDL.[118] The type of carbohydrate in the diet can influence lipoprotein levels, VLDL, in particular. In general, sucrose or fructose in the diet is hyperlipidemic in comparison to glucose or starch. The major changes that follow the metabolism of fructose are increased hepatic synthesis of triglyceride and release of VLDL into the blood in excess of the amounts that can be cleared by peripheral tissues.[108] Increases in the sucrose proportion of the high carbohydrate diet have also resulted in elevated VLDL triglyceride and apo B with increases and decreases in apo B removal being noted.[119]

VI. PROTEIN

In many laboratory animal species, hyperlipidemia results when the semipurified diets contain protein from animal rather than vegetable origin.[120] Several studies in rabbits, in particular, have demonstrated that cholesterol-free diets containing casein as the protein source induces hypercholesterolemia.[121-123] The hypercholesterolemia and/or hypertriglyceridemia in response to casein vs. soy protein diets has also been reported in rats,[124-126] and in pigs.[127] Studies of the protein influence on hypercholes-terolemia have been more variable. For example, in normocholesterolemic individuals several investigations have been unable to demonstrate a significant effect of substitu-tion of soy protein for animal protein on total plasma and lipoprotein cholesterol as well as apo B.[128-130] On the other hand, when hypercholesterolemic individuals were provided with a diet which substituted soy protein for animal protein, significant re-ductions in plasma cholesterol were reported.[131-133] The explanation oftentimes given for the variable effects of casein and soy protein especially in the rabbit is the different lysine:arginine ratio, i.e., 2.0 for the former and 0.9 for the latter.[134] This hypothesis has not been supported in the rat studies.[125] The hypertriglyceridemic response to cas-ein feeding has been attributed to both increased hepatic secretion of VLDL[135] and slower plasma clearance of triglyceride-containing lipoproteins.[126,133,136] Along these lines, studies by Vahoungetal[137] reported that the hyperlipidemia in rats fed a casein-based diet is associated with decreased rates of clearance of chylomicron-like lipopro-teins. Interestingly, in contrast to the earlier rat studies of Sugano et al.[125] the addition of arginine to the casein based diet essentially reversed the delayed clearance observed with casein alone.

VII. ALCOHOL

Ethanol as a dietary component provides approximately 7 kcal/g when oxidized in the body.[138] The caloric contribution of alcohol to the daily energy supply may range at extremes from 0 in teetotalers to 50% in the chronic alcoholic[138] while the ethanol percentage of total calories for the average american diet has been estimated at 7% from dietary recall data in the Multiple Risk Factor Intervention Trial,[139] 6 to 18% for women and 8 to 15% for men in the Lipid Research Clinics Program Prevalance Study,[140] and 3 and 6%, respectively, for women and men in the National Health and Nutrition Examination Survey.[141] Because the major site of degradation of ethanol is the liver which also represents a central organ for lipid-lipoprotein production and catabolism,[142,143] significant alterations in levels of circulating lipids and more subtle changes in lipoprotein metabolism have been documented even with moderate alcohol consumption at 10 to 12% of calories.[143-146] Excessive long-term alcohol intake, on the other hand, results in profound derangements in hepatic lipid metabolism and induc-tion of alcoholic hyperlipemia.[138,142,148]

A. Effect of Ethanol on VLDL and Chylomicron Composition

Although alcoholic hyperlipemia is associated to some extent with increases in all lipoprotein classes,[142,143] elevations in VLDL and plasma triglycerides represent a char-acteristic feature of this disorder which is thus classified as a Type IV hyperlipoprotei-nemia.[142] Interestingly, hyperlipemia prevails at the fatty level stage of alcohol abuse and may represent the attempt of the liver to secrete into circulation rapidly accumu-lating fat stores.[138,142] However, with later stages of liver damage (e.g., cirrhosis) pro-tein export by this organ declines and hyperlipemia may diminish.[142,143] In addition, high levels of dietary fat may exacerbate hypertriglyceridemia in individuals with fatty liver during administration of experimental diets even in the absence of ethanol.[147,148] Since a marked postprandial lipemic response has also been observed in nonalcoholic volunteers given an ethanol bolus along with a fat enriched test meal, the observed hypertriglyceridemia may be the result of synergism between dietary lipid and alcohol.[142]

Plasma phospholipids and cholesterol (primarily nonesterified) are also elevated in individuals with alcoholic hyperlipemia and reflect concurrent elevations in LDL and HDL.[142] However, plasma-free fatty acids are not altered in alcoholics until blood alcohol levels of over 250 mg/dℓ are attained at which point these lipids increase.[142] By contract, short-term ethanol consumption at a level of 7 g/kg/day by swine results in significant decreases in linoleate and increases in palmitic, stearic, and oleic acids esterified to serum triglycerides and phospholipids.[149]

Besides elevations in VLDL, increases in chylomicrons and remnant particles have also been reported in fasted alcoholics.[142,150] However, the extent to which these lipoproteins contribute to elevations in circulating triglyceride in alcoholics is not completely understood.

Following abstinence, plasma triglycerides return to normal levels in chronic alcoholics most rapidly while circulating cholesterol and phospholipids show a slower decline.[142] The appearance of greater amounts of plasma esterified cholesterol during recovery reflects enhanced LCAT activity which may diminish as a result of liver impairment.[142,151]

B. Effect of Ethanol on VLDL and Chylomicron Metabolism

Considerable evidence suggests that alcoholic hyperlipemia may be a response to the increased capacity of liver to synthesize and secrete VLDL.[138,142,143,152] Ethanol metabolism by hepatocytes generates large amounts of NADH which favors synthesis of fatty acids and sn-glycerol-3-phosphate important precursors in triglyceride synthesis.[138,143] Further substrate is provided by increased release and delivery to the liver of fatty acids from peripheral tissue and ethanol induced inhibition of hepatic fatty acid oxidation.[143] These events, along with an alcohol related enhancement in the activity of key enzymes in the triglyceride synthesis pathway, encourage fatty acid esterification and accumulation of triglycerides in hepatocytes.[138,143,152] The presence of excess hepatic triglyceride, along with proliferation of smooth endoplasmic reticulum which accompanies chronic ethanol intake, in turn provides optimal conditions for increased packaging and secretion of VLDL.[138,142,143]

Several pieces of experimental data substantiate that the elevation in plasma lipids following alcohol consumption may result from the above mechanism. First, Triton WR 1339 blockade of VLDL clearance in rats fed ethanol for chronic periods results in the appearance of more serum lipids than in control animals.[142,153] However, this response may vary dramatically depending on ethanol dose.[142,143] Second, incorporation of ^{3}H fatty acid and/or ^{14}C lysine into plasma lipoproteins is increased in humans, rabbits, and rats following administration of alcohol for acute to chronic periods.[142,143] Third, perfused livers[154] and isolated hepatocytes[155] from ethanol fed rats show increased triglyceride and VLDL production. Furthermore, VLDL triglyceride secretion is greatly augmented in ethanol fed baboons with the size of the secreted particles resembling that of chylomicrons.[143] And finally, the VLDL triglyceride synthesis rate estimated from kinetic analyses is significantly elevated in chronic alcoholics.[156]

Although the liver is probably the major production site of VLDL appearing in circulation during alcoholic hyperlipemia,[142,143,157] the intestine may also contribute to the pool of plasma triglyceride following alcohol consumption.[142,143] For example, intraduodenal ethanol infusion in the rat increases the appearance of VLDL in lymph[158] and acute or chronic administration of alcohol enhances labeled fatty acid incorporation into triglyceride in intestinal slices and microsomes.[159] However, alcohol-induced hyperlipemia in rats is prevented following the oral administration of orotic acid which inhibits hepatic but not intestinal triglyceride secretion[160] and hence suggests a minor role for the intestine in the alcohol-lipemic response.[143]

Besides enhanced hepatic VLDL synthesis, an alternative explanation for the appearance of hypertriglyceridemia following chronic ethanol intake is impaired clearance of lipoproteins from circulation.[142,156] Two key enzymes, lipoprotein lipase (LPL) and hepatic triglyceride lipase (HTGL), play an important role in the degradation of triglyceride-rich VLDL and chylomicrons. LPL, located in the capillary endothelium of extrahepatic tissues, degrades the triglyceride core of VLDL and chylomicrons as their surface components are transferred to HDL_3 which is then converted to HDL_2 by the action of LCAT.[156,161,162] HTGL is located on the plasma membranes of hepatic endothelial cells and is responsible for hydrolyzing the phospholipid and triglyceride components of VLDL and chylomicron remnants, HDL_2, and LDL.[142,145,156,163-165] Depending on ethanol dose, acute vs. chronic period of intake, species studied, and degree of liver damage, a wide range of responses has been reported for these two enzymes including no effect, depressed, and accentuated activities.[142,143,156,166,167] For example, HTGL is elevated in alcoholic men with normal liver function but is deficient in individuals with alcoholic hepatitis.[166,168] LPL is increased in chronic alcoholics[166,169] although its activity is depressed in healthy young volunteers during acute ethanol intake at 1 g/kg body weight.[167] More recently, Goldberg et al.[147] demonstrated that acute ingestion of 40 g of alcohol by healthy adult men caused no change in LPL but significantly inhibited HTGL which may thus explain the observed transient elevation in VLDL and HDL in these individuals. By contrast ethanol consumption by nonalcoholics at 24% of calories for a 4-week period did not alter the activity of either enzyme[170] while healthy men who drank 5.5 g of ethanol per kilogram body weight over a 2 1/2-day period had a significant increase in adipose LPL but a substantial decrease in HTGL.[156]

Taskinen et al.[156] have attempted to clarify these time-dose discrepancies by suggesting that acute intake of alcohol may have a transient inhibitory effect on LPL activity which returns to normal levels after 10 hr. Subsequent short-term episodes of drinking enhances LPL activity which is more dramatically increased with prolonged heavy consumption of alcohol.[156,166] The latter may be a compensatory response in the alcoholic to accentuated hepatic VLDL synthesis.[156]

Similarly, acute intake of alcohol may cause a temporary inhibition of HTGL,[145,156] which may later increase in activity in the chronic drinker without evidence of liver dysfunction.[166,171] However, as alcoholic hepatitis develops, a marked depression in HTGL is observed.[169,172]

Other studies have attempted to examine more directly the relationship between ethanol consumption and chylomicron clearance as a possible explanation for alcoholic hyperlipemia.[142,143,173] Acute and chronic alcohol administration to rats does not interfere with the removal of plasma chylomicron triglyceride[142,143] while the clearance of chylomicron cholesteryl ester is significantly delayed.[173] Moreover, acute intake of ethanol by humans impairs chylomicron clearance and decreases HTGL activity[174] while chronic alcohol consumption and associated liver disease lead to a marked depression in HTGL and the appearance of chylomicron remnants in circulation.[143,172]

C. Effect of Ethanol on LDL Composition and Metabolism

As VLDL is degraded by LPL in peripheral tissue, it is first converted to an IDL and finally to LDL.[164] Elevations of the latter in circulation are strongly correlated with the development of coronary heart disease.[175,176] Any ethanol induced alterations in LDL would thus have major pathological implications. Unfortunately, a review of the literature shows that a wide range of responses has been reported for alcohol and this lipoprotein class including no effect,[145,170,177,178] positive,[142,153,156,179-182] and negative[166,183-186] associations. The exact reason for these discrepancies is unclear.

A paucity of information is available concerning the metabolic mechanism(s) responsible for alcohol-related changes in circulating LDL. Moreover, studies showing a depression in LDL cholesterol in alcoholic men have concurrently demonstrated an anomalous increase in precursor VLDL fractional catabolic rate due to enhanced lipoprotein lipase activity.[156,186] On the other hand, we recently observed that the elevated LDL in nonhuman primates fed ethanol at 24% of calories may be the result of increased *de novo* synthesis[187] as well as defective transfer of LDL cholesteryl ester to HDL[181] which would thus result in an enlarged circulating pool of the former.

Finally, although dietary cholesterol plus ethanol at 36% of calories causes an increase in the number of plasma LDL particles in pig-tailed macaques, coronary atherosclerosis is nevertheless reduced in these primates compared to animals fed a cholesterol-enriched diet without ethanol.[179] A possible explanation for the diminished arterial disease is that ethanol may decrease the size, molecular weight, and cholesteryl oleate concentration of the LDL particle which in turn may slow the atherogenic process.[143,179]

D. Ethanol and CHD

Experiments with animals[179,188,189] and a large number of clinical trials[169,185,190-194] have demonstrated that ethanol consumption may reduce the incidence of CHD. Other studies have shown either no effect of ethanol on cholesterol-induced atherosclerosis or a positive association between alcohol intake and cardiovascular disease putatively related to an ethanol-hypertension effect.[142,143,169,195] Chronic heavy alcohol consumption is also associated with stroke, cardiac arrhythmias, and cardiomyopathy.[169,195-197] Thus, some investigators have interpreted this conflicting data to suggest that while moderate drinking, relative to total abstention, may protect against coronary atherosclerosis, excessive ethanol intake may be viewed as a risk factor for CHD.[170]

More recent work has revealed a correlation between the protective effect of alcohol and changes in circulating lipoproteins. Specifically, these studies have shown that moderate alcohol ingestion results in reduced coronary artery occlusion as estimated by coronary angiography, and produces elevations in antiatherogenic HDL.[198-201] On the other hand, drinking patterns may influence this relationship since humans with sporadic intake who consume alcohol in larger amounts at one instance (bout drinking) have more coronary occlusion and lower HDL levels than people who drink consistent amounts of ethanol over time.[201,202]

E. Effect of Ethanol on HDL Composition

An extensive number of studies have shown a positive relationship between moderate alcohol consumption and elevations in HDL lipid and HDLs major protein component, apoprotein A-I.[143,144,156,170,184,185,203-206] Furthermore, one investigator has proposed that HDL cholesterol levels in conjunction with plasma enzymes used to monitor liver function may be a sensitive index of alcohol abuse[203] since alcoholics often have dramatically elevated levels of this lipoprotein class.[166,203,207-210] On the other hand, severe alcoholic hepatitis causes a marked increase in circulating HDL and apoprotein A-I and results in the appearance of an abnormal HDL particle enriched in apoprotein E, phospholipid, and nonesterified cholesterol, and with greatly diminished amounts of cholesteryl ester because of reduced LCAT activity.[142,143,151,211] Moreover, patients with cirrhotic livers have a dramatic depletion in HDL$_3$ which is apparently the nascent lipoprotein particle secreted by the liver.[212]

Upon withdrawal of alcohol from the diet of alcoholic or nonalcoholic subjects,

HDL cholesterol and apoprotein A-I levels decrease significantly and begin to normalize in anywhere from 4 days to 6 weeks depending on the initial level of consumption and/or degree of liver dysfunction.[144,205,207,208] During recovery from alcoholic hepatitis, the HDL_2 subfraction is the first to reappear while HDL_3 returns to the circulation afterward.[151] The former subspecies continues to increase in concentration in these individuals over a 6- to 10-month recovery period.[151] By contrast, transient elevations in HDL can be achieved in as little as 6 hr and reversed in 10 hr in nonalcoholic men given an acute dose of 40 g of ethanol[145] or in 2 1/2 days in normal subjects receiving 160 g/day.[156]

F. Effect of Ethanol on HDL Subfractions

Two major HDL subclasses, HDL_2 (d = 1.063 to 1.125 g/mℓ) and HDL_3 (d = 1.125 to 1.21 g/mℓ), can be distinguished by ultracentrifugation.[213] HDL_2 is the more variable component and is altered by drug therapy, diet, exercise, etc., while the level of HDL_3 is generally less subject to change.[213,214] HDL_3 is the preferred LCAT substrate while HDL_2 may represent the form which protects against coronary artery disease since it is elevated in women and runners[143,144,215,216] but reduced in patients with ischemic heart disease.[213,214] Thus some investigators believe that the HDL_2:HDL_3 ratio is a more sensitive index of coronary risk than the measurement of total HDL.[213,214]

A recent controversy has emerged concerning which HDL subfraction is altered in response to alcohol consumption.[143,144,217] HDL_2 is the major subclass which increases in circulation during acute ethanol intake in normal subjects,[145,156] in alcoholics with minimal or no evidence of liver disease,[164,166,209] and in patients with cirrhotic livers.[212,218] This is also the HDL subfraction which first begins to reappear in the plasma of alcoholics during recovery from severe hepatitis[151] but which decreases dramatically in alcoholics with normal liver function during abstinence.[186] In population studies, HLD_2 is positively correlated with alcohol intake in men while HDL_3 shows this relationship in women.[219] By contrast, Haskell et al.[144] reported that HDL_3 is selectively elevated in men consuming moderate amounts of alcohol and is reduced during abstinence while HDL_2 is refractory to change. Similarly, Williams et al.[220] demonstrated a positive correlation between alcohol consumption and HDL_3 levels in normal adult males while Danielsson et al.[221] showed variable increases in one or the other subclasses in chronic alcoholics with evidence of abnormal liver function.

Lieber[143,217] has attempted to clarify these inconsistencies by suggesting that while moderate alcohol intake is associated with a selective elevation in HDL_3, chronic, high ethanol consumption leads to HDL_2 increases, and alcohol abuse accompanied by extensive liver damage results in diminished levels of both HDL subspecies. While there may be some validity to this scheme, evidence from two studies of alcoholics with cirrhosis indicates that even with severe hepatic dysfunction, HDL_2 levels show a pronounced increase.[212,218] An alternative explanation for these discrepancies in HDL_2 vs. HDL_3 and alcohol consumption may lie in the methodology used to measure these subfractions. All the studies demonstrating elevations in primarily HDL_2 have utilized either high performance liquid chromatography (HPLC) or ultracentrifugation (sequential flotation; density gradient) followed by comprehensive lipid and protein chemical analyses of each HDL subclass.[145,156,164,166,209,212,218] The one population study showing alcohol correlations with either subfraction depending on sex used a two-step precipitation procedure and an indirect measure of HDL_2 cholesterol as the difference between total HDL and HDL_3 cholesterol.[219] The remaining three studies which reported elevations in HDL_3 were carried out using the analytic ultracentrifuge or rate zonal ultracentrifugation where the total mass of HDL fractions was measured from schlieren curves or absorbance at 280 nm instead of analysis of individual lipid and protein components.[144,220,221] Thus, procedural differences may, to a large part, explain some of the discordant HDL subfraction responses to alcohol in the above studies.

G. Effect of Ethanol on HDL Metabolism

A number of animal and human experiments have been performed to determine the metabolic mechanism(s) responsible for the HDL increase as a function of alcohol consumption.[145,153,156,166,171,181,187,211,222-224] Theoretically, ethanol could influence HDLs concentration in circulation by altering the rate of synthesis and secretion, clearance from the plasma compartment, and/or transfer of HDL lipids to LDLs by lipid transfer proteins.[162,181,225] Support for the first mechanism has been widespread because of the well-established induction of hepatic microsomal enzyme activity of ethanol and thus increased capacity for lipoprotein synthesis and secretion.[142,143,204,207,217] This mechanism would favor the production of HDL_3 which is presumably the nascent lipoprotein particle released from the liver.[143,156,166,217] Direct experimental evidence for the enhanced *de novo* synthesis hypothesis comes from in vitro (liver perfusion)[224,226] and in vivo[153] experiments with rats fed alcohol at 36 to 37% of calories which demonstrated increased production of HDL. In addition, we recently showed that squirrel monkeys fed ethanol at 24% of calories incorporate significantly more ^3H mevalonolactone into HDL nonesterified cholesterol in vivo than control animals with the bulk (60%) of the radioactivity appearing in the HDL_3 fraction.[187,222]

Alternatively, elevations in HDL_2 as a function of alcohol consumption may result from enhanced extrahepatic lipoprotein lipase activity which would promote transfer of surface components from VLDL and chylomicrons during lipolysis to nascent HDL_3 particles which are then converted to spherical HDL_2 via the LCAT reaction.[156,161,162,166,171,186] In support of this mechanism, Taskinen et al. reported a marked increase in HDL_2 which correlated with elevated lipoprotein lipase activity in nonalcoholic males during acute ethanol intake[156] and in chronic alcoholics.[166] Other investigators have provided support for this hypothesis by correlating HDL_2 levels in alcoholics with post-heparin plasma lipoprotein lipase activity.[171] Moreover, Sane et al.[186] recently showed that the decreased VLDL fractional catabolic rate which occurs in alcoholics during abstinence correlates with a decline in HDL_2 cholesterol and therefore suggests a relationship between VLDL flux and HDL levels.[162,164,171]

Conversely, alterations in HDL clearance may also contribute to ethanol-related changes in plasma levels of these macromolecules.[145,166,181] HTGL plays an important role in removing HDL_2 from the blood, degrading its lipids, and promoting delivery of HDL to the liver.[145,156,164,165,225] Acute intake of alcohol by health volunteers results in a significant depression in HTGL after 6 to 10 hr followed by a return to normal activity during abstinence[145,156,224] which would thus partially explain any transient increase in HDL_2.[145] However, HTGL activity is increased, although to a lesser extent than LPL, in alcoholic men with normal liver function which may thus accelerate HDL_2 clearance and therefore work counter to the synthesis of HDL promoted by elevated LPL.[166]

Levels of HTGL decrease toward those of nonalcoholics when ethanol is withdrawn from the diet of alcoholics.[166] As might be expected with severe liver damage, HTGL declines markedly[142,169] which may contribute to impaired clearance and the elevated HDL_2 noted in patients with cirrhosis.[212,218] On the other hand, the corresponding decrease in HDL_3 in these individuals may reflect an inability on the part of the liver to synthesize and secrete nascent HDL particles and apoprotein A-I.[170,212]

Other studies using radiolabeled lipoproteins have provided more direct evidence of the effect of ethanol on HDL clearance.[181,211] Nestel et al.[211] determined that the reduced concentrations of HDL and apoprotein A-I seen in alcoholics with hepatitis was the result of a greatly accelerated rate of catabolism. By contrast, we demonstrated that elevations in HDL levels in nonhuman primates fed alcohol at 24% of calories may in part be the result of delayed clearance of these particles from circulation although transfer of cholesteryl ester from HDL to LDLs is apparently not affected by ethanol at this level.[181] Karsenty et al.[225] similarly reported impaired removal of plasma HDL cholesteryl ester in baboons given ethanol at 50% of calories.

VIII. DIETARY FIBER

The influence of dietary fiber on plasma lipids and lipoproteins remains controversial. These conflicting reports have demonstrated that the hypocholesterolemic response of dietary fiber is largely dependent on both the level and type of dietary fiber being consumed. For example, studies by Kay et al.[3] demonstrated reduced plasma cholesterol and triglyceride levels in healthy young men consuming more dietary fiber and fewer fat calories although the issue of which dietary variable was more responsible was raised. On the other hand, Raymond et al.,[230] found no significant changes in plasma cholesterol or triglyceride levels when increased amounts of dietary fiber such as wheat bran, corn and soybean hulls, and cellulose were added to the diets of individuals consuming low and high amounts of cholesterol. Several studies support the importance of the type of fiber used in many investigations. For example, while wheat bran,[231] corn bran,[232] or bagasse (sugar beet)[233] have no significant hypocholesterolemic effect, oat bran[234-236] lowered plasma cholesterol in both normal and hypercholesterolemic individuals. One such study found that consumption of oat bran by hypercholesterolemic men was associated with 13 to 14% reductions in total and LDL cholesterol. Diets containing soybean hulls have also been reported to decrease plasma cholesterol by as much as 14% in healthy individuals.[232]

Preparations of dietary fiber which include pectin,[237,238] lignin,[239] and guar gum[240-242] have been found, in general, to produce a hypocholesterolemic response. Guar gum has been found to be a significantly hypocholesterolemic agent in both normal and Type II hyperlipidemias[240,241] and in one long-term study reduced plasma (15%) and LDL cholesterol (20%) for up to 12 months with no apparent effect on HDL.[242] Studies by Miettinen and Tarpila[243] demonstrated that the 13% reduction in plasma cholesterol in individuals consuming lignin is associated with a 75% increase in fecal bile acids, a mechanism that may be shared by many dietary fibers that have a hypocholesterolemic response. A recent review on dietary fiber[244] summarized the influence that certain fiber-rich foodstuffs have on plasma cholesterol. Thus, apples, carrots, peas, beans, chick peas, and other fruits and vegetables, in general, lower plasma cholesterol, and in particular, LDL cholesterol in man with no significant effect on HDL. This review article also notes that the mechanism(s) of action for the hypocholesterolemic response of dietary fiber remains unclear citing reports of no effect on reduced cholesterol absorption, increased neutral steroid loss and enhanced binding of bile salts.

ACKNOWLEDGMENTS

Preparation of this chapter was made possible through the support of NIH Grant No. HL-23792, HL 34637, NIAA NO. 1 ROI AA06636-01 and the Alcoholic Beverage Medical Research Foundation, The Johns Hopkins University School of Medicine.

The authors express their gratitude to Ms. Kathleen Rourke for her time and effort in the preparation of this chapter.

REFERENCES

1. Gordon, T., Castelli, W. P., Hjortland, M. C., Kannel, W. B., and Dawber, T. R., High density lipoprotein as a protective factor against coronary heart disease, The Framingham study, *Am. J. Med.,* 62, 707, 1977.
2. Wilson, P. W., Garrison, R. J., Castelli, W. P., Feinleib, M., McNamara, P. M., and Kannel, W. B., Prevalence of coronary heart disease in the Framingham Offspring study: study of lipoprotein cholesterols, *Am. J. Cardiol.,* 46, 649, 1980.
3. Miller, G. J. and Miller, N. E., Plasma high density lipoprotein concentration and development of ischaemic heart disease, *Lancet,* 1, 16, 1975.
4. Jenkins, P. J., Harper, R. W., and Nestel, P. J., Severity of coronary atherosclerosis related to lipoprotein concentration, *Br. J. Med.,* 2, 388, 1978.
5. Pownall, H. J., Shepher, J., Mantulin, W. W., Sklar, L. A., and Gotto, A. M., Jr., Effect of saturated and polyunsaturated fat diets on the composition and structure of human low density lipoproteins, *Atherosclerosis,* 36, 299, 1980.
6. Stein, E. A., Shapiro, J., McNerney, C., Glueck, C. J., Tracy, T., et al., Changes in plasma lipid and lipoprotein fractions after alteration in dietary cholesterol, polyunsaturated, saturated and total fat in free-living normal and hypercholesterolemic children, *Am. J. Clin. Nutr.,* 35, 1375, 1982.
7. Ehnholm, C., Huttunen, J. R., Pietinen, P., Leino, U., Mutanen, M., et al., Effect of a diet low in saturated fatty acids on plasma lipids, lipoproteins and HDL subfractions, *Arteriosclerosis,* 4, 265, 1984.
8. Kato, H., Tillotson, J., Nichaman, M. Z., Rhoads, G. G., and Hamilton, H. B., Epidemiological studies of coronary heart disease and stroke in Japanese men living in Japan, Hawaii and California, *Am. J. Epidemiol.,* 97, 372, 1973.
9. Prior, I. A., Davidson, F., Salmond, C. E., and Czochanska, Z., Cholesterol, coconuts, and diets on Polynesian Atolls: a natural experiment: the Pukapuka and Tokelau Island studies, *Am. J. Clin. Nutr.,* 34, 1552, 1981.
10. Shekella, R. B., Shryock, A. M., Paul, O., Leppar, M., Stamler, J., Liu, S., and Raynor, W. J., Jr., Diet, serum cholesterol, and death from coronary heart disease, The Western Electric study, *N. Engl. J. Med.,* 304, 65, 1981.
11. Nichols, A. B., Ravenscroft, C., Lamphiear, D. E., and Ostrander, L. D., Daily nutritional intake and serum lipid levels. The Tecumseh study, *Am. J. Clin. Nutr.,* 29, 1384, 1976.
12. Spritz, N. and Mishkel, M. A., Effects of dietary fats on plasma lipids and lipoproteins: an hypothesis for the lipid lowering effect of unsaturated fatty acids, *J. Clin. Invest.,* 48, 78, 1969.
13. Shepherd, J., Packard, C. J., Grundy, S. M., Yeshurun, D., Gotto, A. M., Jr., and Taunton, O. D., Effects of saturated and polyunsaturated fat diets on the chemical composition and metabolism of low density lipoproteins in man, *J. Lipid Res.,* 21, 91, 1980.
14. Brussard, J. H., Thie-Dallinga, G., Groot, P. H. E., and Katan, M. B., Effects of amount and type of dietary fat on serum lipids, lipoproteins and apolipoproteins in man. A controlled 8-week trial, *Atherosclerosis,* 36, 515, 1980.
15. Vega, G. L., Groszek, E., Wolf, R., and Grundy, S. M., Influence of polyunsaturated fats on composition of plasma lipoproteins and apolipoproteins, *J. Lipid Res.,* 23, 811, 1982.
16. Fless, G. M., Wessler, R. W., and Scanu, A. M., Study of abnormal plasma low density lipoprotein in rhesus monkeys with diet-induced hyperlipidemia, *Biochemistry,* 15, 5799, 1976.
17. Fless, G. M. and Scanu, A. M., Isolation and characterization of the three major low density lipoproteins from normolipidemic rhesus monkeys (*Macaca mulatta*), *J. Biol. Chem.,* 254, 8653, 1979.
18. Rudel, L. L. and Lofland, H. B., Circulating lipoproteins in nonhuman primates, in *Atherosclerosis in Primates,* Vol. 9, Strong, J., Ed., S. Karger, Basel, 224, 1976.
19. Rudel, L. L., Pitts, L. L., and Nelson, C. A., Characterization of plasma low density lipoproteins of nonhuman primates fed dietary cholesterol, *J. Lipid Res.,* 18, 211, 1977.
20. McGill, H. C., Jr., McMahan, C. A., Kruski, A. W., Kelly, J. L., and Mott, G. E., Responses of serum lipoproteins to dietary cholesterol and type of fat in the baboon, *Arteriosclerosis,* 5, 337, 1981.
21. Nelson, C. A. and Morris, M. D., Effects of cholesterol feeding of primate serum lipoproteins. II. Low density lipoprotein characterization from rhesus monkeys with a moderate rise in serum cholesterol, *Biochem. Med.,* 17, 320, 1977.
22. Portman, O. W., Alexander, M., Tanaka, N., and Soltys, P., The effects of dietary fat and cholesterol on the metabolism of plasma low density lipoprotein apoproteins in squirrel monkeys, *Biochem. Biophys. Acta,* 450, 185, 1976.
23. Portman, O. W., Illingworth, D. R., and Alexander, M., The effects of hyperlipidemia on lipoprotein metabolism in squirrel monkeys and rabbits, *Biochem. Biophys. Acta,* 398, 55, 1975.
24. Schonfeld, G., Patsch, W., Rudel, L. L., Nelson, C., Epstein, M., and Olson, R. E., Effect of dietary cholesterol and fatty acids on plasma lipoproteins, *J. Clin. Invest.,* 69, 1072, 1982.

25. Fisher, E. A., Blum, C. B., Zannis, V. I., and Breslow, J. L., Independent effects of dietary saturated fat and cholesterol on plasma lipids, lipoproteins, and apolipoprotein E, *J. Lipid Res.*, 24, 1039, 1983.

26. Turner, J. D., Le, N.-A., and Brown, W. V., Effect of changing dietary fat saturation on low density lipoprotein metabolism in man, *Am. J. Physiol.*, 241, E57, 1981.

27. Nestel, P. J., Billington, T., and Smith, B., Low density and high density lipoprotein kinetics and sterol balance in vegetarians, *Metabolism*, 30, 941, 1981.

28. Vessby, B., Boberg, J., Gustafsson, I. B., Karlstrom, B., Lithell, H., and Ostlund-Lindquist, A. M., Reduction of high density lipoprotein cholesterol and apolipoprotein A-I concentrations by a lipid-lowering diet, *Atherosclerosis*, 35, 21, 1980.

29. Craig, I. H., Phillips, P. J., Lloyd, J. V., Watts, S., Bracken, A., and Read, R., Effects of modified fat diets on LDL/HDL ratio, *Lancet*, ii, 799, 1980.

30. Shepherd, J., Steward, J. M., Clark, J. G., and Carr, K., Sequential changes in plasma lipoproteins and body fat composition during polyunsaturated fat feeding in man, *Br. J. Nutr.*, 44, 265, 1980.

31. Schaefer, E. J., Levy, R. I., Ernst, N. D., Van Sant, F. D., and Brewer, H. B., Jr., The effects of low cholesterol, high polyunsaturated fat, and low-fat diets on plasma lipid and lipoprotein cholesterol levels in normal and hypercholesterolemic subjects, *Am. J. Clin. Nutr.*, 34, 1758, 1981.

32. Nicolosi, R. J., Hojnacki, J. L., Llamsa, N., and Hayes, K. C., Diet and lipoprotein influence on primate atherosclerosis, *Proc. Soc. Exp. Biol. Med.*, 156, 1, 1977.

33. Schwandt, P., Janetschek, P., and Weisweiler, P., High density lipoproteins unaffected by dietary fat modification, *Atherosclerosis*, 44, 9, 1982.

34. Hully, A. V., Cohen, R., and Widdowson, G., Plasma high density lipoprotein cholesterol level — influence of risk factor intervention, *JAMA*, 238, 2269, 1977.

35. Vessby, B., Gustafsson, I. B., Boberg, J., Karlstrom, B., Lithell, H., and Werner, I., Substituting polyunsaturated for saturated fat as a single change in a Swedish diet — effects on serum lipoprotein metabolism and glucose tolerance in patients with hyperlipoproteinemia, *Eur. J. Clin. Invest.*, 10, 193, 1980.

36. Vessby, G., Boberg, J., Gustafsson, I. B., Karlstrom, B., Lithwell, H., and Ostlund-Lindquist, A. M., Reduction of high density lipoprotein cholesterol apolipoprotein A-I concentrations by a lipid-lowering diet, *Atherosclerosis*, 35, 21, 1980.

37. Parks, J. S. and Rudel, L. L., Different kinetic fates of apolipoproteins A-I and A-II from lymph chylomicra of nonhuman primates. Effect of saturated versus polyunsaturated dietary fat, *J. Lipid Res.*, 23, 410, 1982.

38. Shepherd, J., Packard, C. J., Patsch, J. R., Gotto, A. M., Jr., and Taunton, O. D., Effects of dietary polyunsaturated and saturated fat on the properties of high density lipoproteins and the metabolism of apolipoprotein A-I, *J. Clin. Invest.*, 61, 1582, 1978.

39. Oster, P., Schlierf, G., Heuck, C. C., Hahn, S., Szymanski, and Schellenberg, B., Diet and high density lipoproteins, *Lipids*, 16, 93, 1981.

40. Chait, A., Onitiri, A., Nicoll, A., Rabaya, E., Davies, J., and Lewis, B., Reduction of serum triglyceride levels by polyunsaturated fat, *Atherosclerosis*, 20, 347, 1974.

41. Hjermann, I., Enger, S. C., Helgeland, A., Holme, I., Leven, P., and Trygg, K., The effect of dietary changes on high density lipoprotein cholesterol. The Oslo study, *Am. J. Med.*, 66, 105, 1979.

42. Lock, D. R., Varhol, A., Grimes, S., Patsch, W., and Schonfeld, G., Apo A-I/Apo A-II ratios in plasma of vegetarians, *Metabolism*, 32, 1142, 1983.

43. Lasser, N. L., Roheim, P. S., Edelstein, D., and Eder, H. A., Serum lipoproteins of normal and cholesterol-fed rats, *J. Lipid Res.*, 14, 1, 1973.

44. Mahley, R. W., Weisgraber, K. H., Innerarity, T., Brewer, H. B., Jr., and Assman, G., Swine lipoproteins and atherosclerosis: changes in the plasma lipoproteins and apoproteins induced by cholesterol feedings, *Biochemistry*, 14, 2817, 1975.

45. Mahley, R. W., Weisgraber, K. H., and Innerarity, T. L., Canine lipoproteins and atherosclerosis. II. Characterization of the plasma lipoproteins associated with atherogenic and nonatherogenic hyperlipidemia, *Circ. Res.*, 35, 722, 1974.

46. Kuehl, K. S., Roheim, P. S., Wolinsky, H., and Eder, H. A., Serum lipoproteins in normal and cholesterol fed monkeys, *Circulation*, 50, 94, 1974.

47. Rudel, L. L., Shah, R., and Greene, D. G., Study of the atherogenic dyslipoproteinemia induced by dietary cholesterol in rhesus monkeys (*Macaca mulatta*), *J. Lipid Res.*, 20, 55, 1979.

48. Chong, K. S., Nicolosi, R. J., Rodger, R. F., Arrigo, D. A., Yuan, R. W., Mackey, J. J., and Herbert, P. N., Effect of dietary fat saturation on plasma lipoproteins and high density lipoprotein metabolism of the rhesus monkey, submitted, 1986.

49. Rudel, L. L. and Pitts, L. L., Male-female variability in the dietary cholesterol-induced hyperlipoproteinemia of cynomolgus monkeys (*Macaca fascicularis*), *J. Lipid Res.*, 19, 992, 1978.

50. Kushwaha, R. S., Foster, D. M., and Hazzard, W. R., Effect of diet-induced hypercholesterolemia on high density lipoprotein metabolism in pigtail monkeys (*Macaca nemestrina*), *Metabolism,* 31, 43, 1982.
51. Srinivasan, S. R., Radhakrishnanurthy, B., Smith, C. C., Wolf, R. H., and Berenson, G. S., Serum lipid and lipoprotein responses of six nonhuman primate species to dietary changes in cholesterol levels, *J. Nutr.,* 106, 1757, 1976.
52. Rudel, L. L., Reynold, J. A., Bullock, B. C., Nutritional effects on blood lipid and HDL cholesterol concentrations in two subspecies of African Green monkeys (*Cercopithecus aethiops*), *J. Lipid Res.,* 22, 278, 1981.
53. Cole, T. G., Patsch, W., Kuisk, I., Gonen, B., and Schonfeld, Increases in dietary cholesterol and fat raise levels of apolipoprotein E-containing lipoproteins in the plasma of man, *J. Clin. Endocrinol. Metab.,* 56, 1108, 1978.
54. Mahley, R. W., Innerarity, T. L., Bersot, T. P., Lipson, A., and Margolis, S., Alterations in human high density lipoproteins, with or without increased plasma cholesterol, induced by diets high in cholesterol, *Lancet,* 2, 807, 1978.
55. Danielsson, B., Ekman, R., Johansson, B. G., Nilsson-Ehle, P., and Petersson, B. G., Isolation of a high density lipoprotein with high contents of arginine-rich apoprotein (apo E) from rat plasma, *FEBS Lett.,* 86, 299, 1978.
56. Weisgraber, K. H., Mahley, R. W., and Assman, G., Identification of the rat arginine-rich apoprotein and its redistribution following injection of iodinated lipoproteins into normal and hypercholesterolemic rats, *Atherosclerosis,* 28, 121, 1977.
57. Innerarity, T. L., Pitas, R. E., and Mahley, R. W., Disparities in the interaction of rat and human lipoproteins with cultured rat fibroblasts and smooth muscle cells, *J. Biol. Chem.,* 255, 11163, 1980.
58. Mahley, R. W., Alterations in plasma lipoproteins induced by cholesterol feeding in animals including man, in *Disturbances in Lipid and Lipoprotein Metabolism,* Dietschy, J. M., Gotto, A. M., Jr., and Ontko, J. A., Eds., American Physiological Society, Bethesda, Md., 1978, 181.
59. Mahley, R. W., Atherogenic hyperlipoproteinemia: the cellular and molecular biology of plasma lipoproteins altered by dietary fat and cholesterol, in *Medical Clinics of North America: Lipid Disorders,* Vol. 66, Havel, R. J., Ed., W. B. Saunders, Philadelphia, 1982, 375.
60. Lin-Lee, Y. C., Tanaka, Y., Lin, C. T., and Chan, L., Effects of an atherogenic diet on apolipoprotein E biosynthesis in the rat, *Biochemistry,* 20, 6474, 1981.
61. Kris-Etherton, P. M. and Cooper, A. D., Studies on the etiology of the hyperlipemia in rats fed an atherogenic diet, *J. Lipid Res.,* 21, 435, 1980.
62. Reitman, J. S. and Mahley, R. W., Yucatan miniature swine lipoproteins: changes induced by cholesterol feeding, *Biochem. Biophys. Acta,* 575, 446, 1979.
63. Shore, V. G., Shore, B., and Hart, R. G., Changes in apolipoproteins and properties of rabbit very low density lipoproteins on induction of cholesterolemia, *Biochemistry,* 13, 1579, 1974.
64. Mahley, R. W., Weisgraber, K. H., and Innerarity, T., Atherogenic hyperlipoproteinemia induced by cholesterol feeding in the Patas monkey, *Biochemistry,* 15, 2979, 1976.
65. Fox, J., Carey, R. D., McGill, H., and Getz, G., Hepatic apolipoprotein apo A-I mRNA levels in baboons fed cholesterol and polyunsaturated fat or saturated fat, *Arteriosclerosis,* 4, 561a, 1984.
66. Sorci-Thomas, M., Stockbine, P., Rudel, L. L., and Williams, D. L., Regulation of apolipoprotein A-I mRNA levels by dietary fat and cholesterol, *Arteriosclerosis,* 5, 5329, 1985.
67. Phillipson, B. E., Rothrock, D. W., Connor, W. E., Harris, W. S., and Illingworth, D. R., Reduction of plasma lipids, lipoproteins, and apoproteins by dietary fish oils in patients with hypertriglyceridemia, *N. Engl. J. Med.,* 312, 1210, 1985.
68. McKee, G., Eicosapentaenoic acid and coronary heart disease, in *Nutrition and the M.D.,* Vol. 3, Publisher PM, Van Nuys, Calif., 1983, 3.
69. Glomset, J. A., Fish, fatty acids, and human health, *N. Engl. J. Med.,* 312, 1253, 1985.
70. Medical News: It's not fishy; fruit of the sea may foil cardiovascular disease, *JAMA,* 247, 729, 1982.
71. Bang, H. O., Dyerberg, J., and Nielsen, A. B., Plasma lipid and lipoprotein pattern in Greenland west coast Eskimos, *Lancet,* 1, 1143, 1971.
72. Bang, H. O. and Dyerberg, J., Plasma lipids and lipoproteins in Greenlanoic west coast Eskimos, *Acta Med. Scand.,* 192, 85, 1972.
73. Balasubramaniam, S., Simons, L. A., Chang, S., and Hickie, J. B., Reduction in plasma cholesterol by a diet rich in n-3 fatty acids in the rat, *J. Lipid Res.,* 26, 634, 1985.
74. Sanders, T. A. B., Vickers, M., and Haines, A. P., Effect on blood lipids and haemostasis of a supplement of cod-liver oil, rich in eicosopentaenoic and docosanexaenoic acids, in healthy young men, *Clin. Sci.,* 61, 317.
75. Bronsgest-Schoute, H. C., van Gent, C. M., Luten, J. B., and Ruiter, A., The effect of various intakes of omega 3-fatty acids on the blood lipid composition in healthy human subjects, *Am. J. Clin. Nutr.,* 34, 1752, 1981.

76. Von Lossonczy, T. O., Ruiter, A., Bronsgeest-Schoute, H. C., van Gent, C. M., and Hermus, R. J. J., The effect of a fish diet on serum lipids in healthy human subjects, *Am. J. Clin. Nutr.*, 31, 1340, 1978.
77. Reed, S. A., Dietary source of ω-3-eicosapentaenoic acid, *Lancet*, 2, 739, 1979.
78. Dyerberg, J., Bang, H. O., and Stoffersen, E., Eicosapentaenoic acid and prevention of thrombosis and atherosclerosis?, *Lancet*, 2, 117, 1978.
79. Harris, W. S., Connor, W. E., and McMurry, M. P., The comparative reductions of the plasma lipids and lipoproteins by dietary polyunsaturated fats: salmon oil versus vegetable oils, *Metabolism*, 32, 179, 1983.
80. Dyerberg, J., Bang, H. O., and Hjorne, N., Fatty acid composition of the plasma lipids in Greenland Eskimos, *Am. J. Clin. Nutr.*, 28, 958, 1975.
81. Culp, B. R., Lands, W. E. M., Lucches, B. R., Pitt, R., and Romson, J., The effect of dietary supplementation of fish oil on experimental myocardial infarction, *Prostaglandins*, 20, 1021, 1980.
82. Brockerhoff, H., Hoyle, R. J., and Huang, P. C., Incorporation of fatty acids of marine origin into triglycerides and phospholipids of mammals, *Biochim. Biophys. Acta*, 144, 541, 1967.
83. Harris, W. S., Connor, W. E., Inkeles, S. B., and Illingworth, D. R., Dietary omega-3 fatty acids prevent carbohydrate-induced hypertriglyceridemia, *Metabolism*, 33, 1016, 1984.
84. Kingsbury, K. J., Aylott, C., Morgan, D. M., and Emmerson, R., Effects of ethyl arachidonate, cod-liver oil, and corn oil on the plasma-cholesterol level, *Lancet*, 1, 739, 1961.
85. Peifer, J. J., Lundbury, W. O., Ishio, S., and Warmanen, E., Changes in hypercholesteremia and tissue fatty acids induced by dietary fats and marine oil fractions, *Arch. Biochem. Biophys.*, 110, 270, 1985.
86. Harris, W. S. and Connor, W. E., The effect of salmon oil upon plasma lipids, lipoproteins, and triglyceride clearance, *Trans. Assoc. Am. Physicians*, 43, 148, 1980.
87. Kinsell, L. W., Michaels, G. D., Walker, G., and Visintine, R. E., The effect of a fish-oil fraction on plasma lipids, *Diabetes*, 10, 316, 1961.
88. Fehily, A. M., Burr, M. L., Phillips, K. M., and Deadman, N. M., The effect of fatty fish on plasma lipid and lipoprotein concentrations, *Am. J. Clin. Nutr.*, 38, 349, 1983.
89. Nestel, P. J., Connor, W. E., Reardon, M. F., Connor, S., Wong, S., and Boston, R., Suppression by diets rich in fish oil of very low density lipoprotein production in man, *J. Clin. Invest.*, 74, 82, 1984.
90. Yarnell, J. W. G., Milbank, J., Walker, C. L., Fehily, A. M., and Hayes, T. M., Determinants of high density lipoprotein and total cholesterol in women, *J. Epidemiol. Commun. Health*, 36, 167, 1982.
91. Illingworth, D. R., Harris, W. S., and Connor, W. E., Inhibition of low density lipoprotein synthesis by dietary omega-3 fatty acids in humans, *Arteriosclerosis*, 4, 270, 1984.
92. Saynor, R. and Verel, D., Eskimos and their diets, *Lancet*, 1, 1335, 1983.
93. Kromhout, D., Bosschieter, E. B., and Coulander, C. L., The inverse relation between fish consumption and 20-year mortality from coronary heart disease, *N. Engl. J. Med.*, 312, 1205, 1985.
94. Sanders, T. A. B. and Younger, K. M., The effect of dietary supplements of omega-3 polyunsaturated fatty acids on the fatty acid composition of platelets and plasma choline phosphoglycerides, *Br. J. Nutr.*, 45, 613—616.
95. Yang, Y. T. and Williams, M. A., Comparison of C_{18}-, C_{20}-, and C_{22}-unsaturated fatty acids in reducing fatty acid synthesis in isolated rat hepatocytes, *Biochim. Biophys. Acta*, 531, 133, 1978.
96. Wong, S. H., Nestel, P. J., Trimble, R. P., Storer, G. B., Illman, R. J., and Topping, D. L., The adaptive effects of dietary fish and safflower oil on lipid and lipoprotein metabolism in perfused rat liver, *Biochim. Biophys. Acta*, 792, 103, 1984.
97. Iritani, N., Fukuda, E., Inoguchi, K., Tsubosaka, M., and Tashiro, S., Reduction of lipogenic enzymes by shellfish triglycerides in rat liver, *J. Nutr.*, 110, 1664, 1980.
98. Grundy, S. M., Ahrens, E. H., and Mhettinen, T. A., Quantitative isolation and gas-liquid chromatographic analysis of total fecal bile acids, *J. Lipid Res.*, 6, 397, 1965.
99. Connor, W. E., Lin, D. S., and Harris, W. S., A comparison of dietary polyunsaturated omega-6 and omega-3 fatty acids in humans: effects upon plasma lipids, lipoproteins and sterol balance, *Arteriosclerosis*, 1, 363a, 1981.
100. Chen, I. S., Subramaniam, S., Cassidy, M. M., Sheppard, A. J., and Vahouny, G. V., Intestinal absorption and lipoprotein transport of (omega-3) eicosapentaenoic acid, *J. Nutr.*, 115, 219, 1985.
101. Botting, N. R., Vandenberg, G. A., and Reiser, R., Resistance of certain long-chain polyunsaturated fatty acids of marine oils to pancreatic lipase hydrolysis, *Lipids*, 2, 489, 1967.
102. Gavigan, S. J. P. and Knight, B. L., Catabolism of low density lipoprotein by fibroblasts cultured in media supplemented with saturated or unsaturated free fatty acids, *Biochem. Biophys. Acta*, 668, 632, 1981.

103. Sanders, T. A. B. and Roshanai, F., The influence of different types of omega-3 polyunsaturated fatty acids on blood lipids and platelet function in healthy volunteers, *Clin. Sci.*, 64, 91, 1983.
104. Sanders, T. A. B., Sullivan, D. R., Reeve, J., and Thompson, G. R., Triglyceride-lowering effect of marine polyunsaturates in patients with hypertriglyceridemia, *Arteriosclerosis*, 5, 459, 1985.
105. Watkins, D. M., Froeb, H. F., Hatch, F. T., and Gutman, A. B., Effects of diet in essential hypertension. II. Results with unmodified Kempner rice diet in 50 fully hospitalized patients, *Am. J. Med.*, 9, 441, 1950.
106. Ahrens, E. H., Jr., Hirsch, J., Oette, K., Farquhar, J. W., and Stein, Y., Carbohydrate-induced and fat-induced lipemia, *Trans. Assoc. Am. Physicians*, 74, 134, 1961.
107. Antonis, A. and Bersohn, I., The influence of diet on serum triglycerides in South African White and Bantu prisoners, *Lancet*, 1, 3, 1961.
108. Little, J. A., McGuire, V., and Derksen, A., Available carbohydrates, in *Nutrition, Lipids, and Coronary Heart Disease*, Vol. 1, Levy, R. I., Rifkind, B. M., Dennis, B. H., and Ernest, N., Eds., Raven Press, New York, 1979, 119.
109. Quarfordt, S. H., Frank, A., Shames, D. M., Berman, M., and Steinberg, D., Very low density lipoprotein triglyceride transport in type IV hyperlipoproteinemia and the effects of carbohydrate-rich diets, *J. Clin. Invest.*, 49, 2281, 1970.
110. Vessby, B. and Carlson, L. A., Conversion of type III hyperlipoproteinemia to type IV hyperlipoproteinemia by a fat-free, carbohydrate-rich diet, *Eur. J. Clin. Invest.*, 5, 359, 1975.
111. Grundy, S. M. and Mok, H. Y., Chylomicron clearance in normal and hyperlipidemic man, *Metabolism*, 25, 1225, 1976.
112. Hegsted, D. M., McGandy, R. B., Myers, M. L., and Stare, F. J., Quantitative effects of dietary fat on serum cholesterol in man, *Am. J. Clin. Nutr.*, 17, 281, 1965.
113. Gonen, B., Patsch, W., Kuisk, I., and Schonfeld, G., The effect of short-term feeding of a high carbohydrate diet on HDL subclasses in normal subjects, *Metabolism*, 30, 1125, 1981.
114. Schonfeld, G., Weidman, S. W., Witztum, J. L., and Bowman, R. M., Alterations in levels and interrelations of plasma apolipoproteins induced by diet, *Metabolism*, 25, 261, 1976.
115. Kashyap, M. L., Barnhart, R. L., Srivastana, L. S., Perisutti, G., Vink, P., et al., Effects of dietary carbohydrate and fat on plasma lipoproteins and apolipoproteins CII and CIII in healthy men, *J. Lipid Res.*, 23, 877, 1982.
116. Blum, C. B., Levy, R. I., Eisenberg, S., Hall, M., Goebal, R. H., et al., High density lipoprotein metabolism in man, *J. Clin. Invest.*, 60, 795, 1977.
117. Quarfordt, S. H., Michalopoulos, G., and Schirmer, B., The effect of human C apolipoproteins on the *in vitro* hepatic metabolism of triglyceride emulsions in the rat, *J. Biol. Chem.*, 257, 1982.
118. Huff, M. W. and Nestel, P. J., Metabolism of apolipoproteins CII, CIII, $CIII_2$ and VLDL-B in human subjects consuming high carbohydrate diets, *Metabolism*, 31, 493, 1982.
119. Nestel, P. J., Reardon, M., and Fidge, N. H., Sucrose induced changes in VLDL and LDL-B apoprotein removal rates, *Metabolism*, 28, 531, 1979.
120. Carroll, K. K., The role of dietary protein in hypercholesterolemia and atherosclerosis, *Lipids*, 13, 360, 1978.
121. Kritchevsky, D., Vegetable protein and atherosclerosis, *J. Am. Oil Chem. Soc.*, 56, 135, 1979.
122. Hamilton, R. M. G. and Carroll, K. K., Plasma cholesterol levels in rabbits fed low fat, low cholesterol diets — effects of dietary proteins, carbohydrates and fiber from different sources, *Atherosclerosis*, 24, 47, 1976.
123. Terpstra, A. H. M., Harkes, L., and Van der Veen, F. H., The effect of different proportions of casein in semipurified diets on the concentration of serum cholesterol and lipoprotein composition in rabbits, *Lipids*, 16, 114, 1981.
124. Nagata, Y., Ishikawa, N., and Sugano, M., Studies of the mechanism of antihypercholesterolemic action of soy protein and soy-protein type amino acid mixture in relationship to casein counterparts in rats, *J. Nutr.*, 112, 1614, 1982.
125. Sugano, M., Ishikawa, N., Nagata, Y., and Imaizumi, K., Effect of arginine and lysine additions to casein and soy-bean protein on serum lipid, apolipoproteins, insulin and glucagon in rats, *Br. J. Nutr.*, 48, 211, 1982.
126. Cohn, J. S., Krimpton, W. G., and Nestel, P. J., The effect of dietary casein and soy protein on cholesterol and very low density lipoprotein metabolism in the rat, *Atherosclerosis*, 52, 219, 1984.
127. Kim, D. N., Lee, K. T., Reiner, J. M., and Thomas, W. A., Effects of soy protein on cholesterol metabolism in swine, in *Animal and Vegetable Proteins in Lipid Metabolism and Atherosclerosis*, Gibney, M. J. and Kritchevsky, D., Eds., Alan R. Liss, New York, 1983, 101.
128. Grundy, S. M. and Abrams, J. J., Comparison of actions of soy protein and casein on metabolism of plasma lipoproteins and cholesterol in humans, *Am. J. Clin. Nutr.*, 38, 245, 1983.

129. Goldberg, A. P., Lim, A., Kolar, J. B., Grundhauser, J. J., Steinke, F. H., et al., Soybean protein independently lowers plasma cholesterol levels in primary hypercholesterolemia, *Atherosclerosis,* 43, 355, 1982.

130. Sacks, F. M., Breslow, J. L., Wood, P. G., and Kass, E. H., Lack of an effect of dairy protein (casein) and soy protein on plasma cholesterol of strict vegetarians, *J. Lipid Res.,* 24, 101, 1983.

131. Descovich, G. C., Ceredi, C., Gaddi, A., Benassi, M. S., Mannino, G., et al., Multicentre study of soybean protein diet for outpatient hypercholesterolemic patients, *Lancet,* 2, 709, 1980.

132. Sirtori, C. R., Gatti, E., Mantero, O., Conti, F., Agradi, E., Tremoli, E., Sirtori, M., Fratterrigo, L., Travazzi, L., and Kritchevsky, D., Clinical experience with the soybean protein diet in treatment of hypercholesterolemia, *Am. J. Clin. Nutr.,* 32, 1645, 1979.

133. Huff, M. W., Giovanetti, P. M., and Wolfe, B. M., Turnover of very low density lipoprotein-apoprotein B is increased by substitution of soybean protein for meat and dairy protein in the diets of hypercholesterolemic men, *Am. J. Clin. Nutr.,* 39, 888, 1984.

134. Kritchevsky, D., Tepper, S. A., Czarnecki, S. K., and Klurfeld, D. M., Atherogenicity of animal and vegetable protein, *Atherosclerosis,* 41, 42917, 1982.

135. Sugano, M., Tanaka, K., and Ide, T., Secretion of cholesterol and triglycerides and apolipoprotein A-I by isolated perfused liver from rats fed soy bean protein and casein or their amino acid mixtures, *J. Nutr.,* 112, 855, 1982.

136. Roberts, D. C. K., Stalmbach, M. E., Khalil, M. W., Hutchinson, J. C., and Carroll, K. K., Effects of dietary protein on composition and turnover of apoproteins in plasma lipoprotein of rabbits, *Can. J. Biochem.,* 56, 642, 1981.

137. Vahouny, G. V., Adamson, I., Chalcarz, W., Satchithanandam, S., Meusing, R., Klurfeld, D. M., Tepper, S. A., Saughui, A., and Kritchersky, D., Effects of casein and soy protein on hepatic and serum lipids and lipoprotein distributions in the rat, *Atherosclerosis,* 56, 127, 1958.

138. Lieber, C. S., The metabolism of alcohol, *Sci. Am.,* 243, 25, 1976.

139. LaPorte, R., Valvo-Gerard, L., Kuller, L., Dai, W., Bates, M., Cresanta, J., Williams, K., and Palkin, D., The relationship between alcohol consumption, liver enzymes and high-density lipoprotein cholesterol, *Circulation,* 64, 67, 1981.

140. Dennis, B. H., Haynes, S. G., Anderson, J., Liu-Chi, S,. Hosking, J. D., and Rifkind, B. M., Nutrient intakes among selected North American populations in the Lipid Research Clinics Prevalence study: composition of energy intake, *Am. J. Clin. Nutr.,* 41, 312, 1985.

141. Gruchow, H. W., Sobocinski, K. A., Baboriak, J. J., and Schelter, J. G., Alcohol consumption, nutrient intake and relative body weight among U.S. adults, *Am. J. Clin. Nutr.,* 42, 289, 1985.

142. Baraona, E. and Lieber, C. S., Effects of ethanol on lipid metabolism, *J. Lipid Res.,* 20, 289, 1979.

143. Lieber, C. S. and Savolainen, M., Ethanol and lipids, alcoholism, *Clin. Exp. Res.,* 8, 409, 1984.

144. Haskell, W. L., Camargo, C., Williams, P. T., Vranizan, K. M., Krauss, R. M., Lindgren, F. T., and Wood, P. D., The effect of cessation and resumption of moderate alcohol intake on serum high-density lipoprotein subfractions, *N. Engl. J. Med.,* 310, 805, 1984.

145. Goldberg, C. S., Tall, A. R., and Krumholz, S., Acute inhibition of hepatic lipase and increase in plasma lipoproteins after alcohol intake, *J. Lipid Res.,* 25, 714, 1984.

146. Mulligan, J. J., Cluette-Brown, J. E., Noring, R., Igoe, F. D., Chong, J., and Hojnacki, J. L., Effect of ethanol on lecithin:cholesterol acyltransferase (LCAT) activity, *Res. Commun. Chem. Pathol. Pharmacol.,* 47, 181, 1985.

147. Borosky, S. A., Perlow, W., Baraona, E., and Lieber, C. S., Relationship of alcoholic hypertriglyceridemia to stage of liver disease and dietary lipid, *Dig. Dis. Sci.,* 25, 22, 1980.

148. Avgerinos, A., Chu, P., Greenfield, C., Harry, I. S., and McIntyre, N., Plasma lipid and lipoprotein response to fat feeding in alcoholic liver disease, *Hepatology,* 3, 349, 1983.

149. Foudin, L., Tumbleson, M. E., Sun, A. Y., Geister, R. W., and Sun, G. Y., Ethanol consumption and serum lipid profiles in Sinclair (S-1) miniature swine, *Life Sci.,* 34, 819, 1983.

150. Chait, A., Mancini, M., February, A. W., and Lewis, B., Clinical and metabolic study of alcoholic hyperlipemia, *Lancet,* 2, 62, 1972.

151. Weidman, S. W., Ragland, J. B., and Sabesin, S. M., Plasma lipoprotein composition in alcoholic hepatitis: accumulation of apolipoprotein E-rich high density lipoprotein and preferential reappearance of "light"-HDL during partial recovery, *J. Lipid Res.,* 23, 556, 1982.

152. Savolainen, M. J., Baraona, E., Pikkarainen, P., and Lieber, C. S., Hepatic triacylglycerol synthesizing activity during progression of alcoholic liver injury in the baboon, *J. Lipid Res.,* 25, 813, 1984.

153. Baraona, E. and Lieber, C. S., Effects of chronic ethanol feeding on serum lipoprotein metabolism in the rat, *J. Clin. Invest.,* 49, 769, 1970.

154. Morland, J. and Oye, I., Effect of acute and chronic ethanol treatment on hepatic triglyceride release from the rat perfused liver, *Eur. J. Pharmacol.,* 27, 238, 1974.

155. Lakshmanan, M. R., Felver, M. E., and Veech, R. L., Alcohol and VLDL synthesis and secretion by isolated hepatocytes, alcoholism, *Clin. Exp. Res.,* 4, 361, 1980.

156. Taskinen, M., Valimaki, M., Nikkila, E. A., Kuusi, T., and Ylikahri, R., Sequence of alcohol-induced initial changes in plasma lipoproteins (VLDL and HDL) and lipolytic enzymes in humans, *Metabolism*, 34, 112, 1985.

157. Lakshmanan, M. R., Felver, M. E., and Ezekiel, M., Relationship of endocrine status on the stimulatory effect of ethanol on hepatic very low density lipoprotein synthesis, alcoholism, *Clin. Exp. Res.*, 8, 359, 1984.

158. Mistilis, S. P. and Ockner, R. K., Effects of ethanol on endogenous lipid and lipoprotein metabolism in small intestine, *J. Lab. Clin. Med.*, 80, 34, 1972.

159. Carter, E. A., Dummey, G. D., and Isselbacher, K. J., Ethanol stimulates triglyceride synthesis by the intestine, *Science*, 174, 1245, 1971.

160. Hernell, O. and Johnson, O., Effects of ethanol on plasma triglycerides in male and female rats, *Lipids*, 8, 503, 1973.

161. Dieplinger, H., Zechner, R., and Kostner, G. M., The in vitro formation of HDL_2 during the action of LCAT: the role of triglyceride-rich lipoproteins, *J. Lipid Res.*, 26, 273, 1985.

162. Tall, A. R. and Small, D. M., Plasma high-density lipoproteins, *N. Engl. J. Med.*, 22, 1232, 1978.

163. Grosser, J., Schrecker, O., and Greten, H., Function of hepatic triglyceride lipase in lipoprotein metabolism, *J. Lipid Res.*, 22, 437, 1981.

164. Nilsson-Ehle, P., Garfinkel, A. S., and Schotz, M. C., Lipolytic enzymes and plasma lipoprotein metabolism, *Ann. Rev. Biochem.*, 49, 667, 1980.

165. Bamberger, M., Glick, J. M., and Rothblat, G. H., Hepatic lipase stimulates the uptake of high density lipoprotein cholesterol by hepatoma cells, *J. Lipid Res.*, 24, 869, 1983.

166. Taskinen, M., Valimaki, M., Nikkila, E. A., Kuusi, T., Ehnholm, C., and Ylikahri, R., High density lipoprotein subfractions and postheparin plasma lipases in alcoholic men before and after ethanol withdrawal, *Metabolism*, 31, 1168, 1982.

167. Nilsson-Ehle, P., Carlstrom, S., Belfrage, P., Effects of ethanol intake on lipoprotein lipase activity in adipose tissue of fasting subjects, *Lipids*, 13, 433, 1978.

168. Freeman, M., Kuiden, L., Ragland, J. B., and Sabesin, S. M., Hepatic triglyceride lipase deficiency in liver disease, *Lipids*, 12, 443, 1977.

169. Devenyi, P., Robinson, G. M., and Roncari, D. A. K., Alcohol and high-density lipoproteins, *J. Can. Med. Assoc.*, 123, 981, 1980.

170. Crouse, J. R. and Grundy, S. M., Effect of alcohol on plasma lipoproteins and cholesterol and triglyceride metabolism in man, *J. Lipid Res.*, 25, 486, 1984.

171. Ekman, R., Fex, G., Johansson, B. G., Nilsson-Ehle, P., and Wastein, J., Changes in plasma high density lipoproteins and lipolytic enzymes after long-term, heavy ethanol consumption, *Scand. J. Clin. Lab. Invest.*, 41, 709, 1981.

172. Muller, P., Fellin, R., and Lamprecht, J., Hypertriglyceridemia secondary to liver disease, *Eur. J. Clin. Lab. Invest.*, 4, 419, 1974.

173. Redgrave, T. G. and Martin, G., Effects of chronic ethanol consumption on the catabolism of chylomicron triacylglycerol and cholesteryl ester in the rat, *Atherosclerosis*, 28, 69, 1977.

174. Schneider, J., Panne, E., Braun, H., Mordasini, R., and Kaffarnik, H., Ethanol-induced hyperlipoproteinemia. Crucial role of preceding ethanol intake in the removal of chylomicrons, *J. Lab. Clin. Med.*, 101, 114, 1983.

175. Levy, R. I., Cholesterol, lipoproteins, apoproteins and heart disease: present status and future prospects, *Clin. Chem.*, 27, 653, 1981.

176. Packard, C. J. and Shepherd, J., Low-density lipoprotein receptor pathway in man: its role in regulating plasma low-density lipoprotein levels, in *Atherosclerosis Reviews*, Vol. 2, Grotto, A. M. and Paoletti, R., Eds., Raven Press, New York, 1983, 29.

177. Topping, D. L., Weller, R. A., Nadar, C. J., Calvert, G. D., and Illman, R. J., Adaptive effects of dietary ethanol in the pig: changes in plasma high-density lipoproteins and fecal steroid excretion and mutagenicity, *Am. J. Clin. Nutr.*, 36, 245, 1982.

178. Stamford, B. A., Mattler, S., Fell, R. D., Sady, S., Cresanta, M. K., and Papanek, P., Cigarette smoking, physical activity, and alcohol consumption: relationship to blood lipids and lipoproteins in premenopausal females, *Metabolism*, 33, 585, 1984.

179. Rudel, L. L., Leathers, C. W., Bond, M. G., and Bullock, B. C., Dietary ethanol-induced modifications in hyperlipoproteinemia and atherosclerosis in nonhuman primates, (*Macaca nemestrina*), *Arteriosclerosis*, 1, 144, 1981.

180. Glueck, C. J., Heiss, G., Morrison, J. A., Khoury, P., and Moore, M., Alcohol intake, cigarette smoking and plasma lipids and lipoproteins in 12- to 19-year-old children, *Circulation*, 64, 48, 1981.

181. Cluette-Brown, J., Mulligan, J., Igoe, F., Doyle, K., and Hojnacki, J., Ethanol induced alterations in low and high density lipoproteins, *Proc. Soc. Exp. Biol. Med.*, 178, 495, 1985.

182. Shepherd, R. J., Cox, M., and West, C., Some factors influencing serum lipid levels in a working population, *Atherosclerosis*, 35, 287, 1980.

183. Mezey, E., Metabolic effects of alcohol, *Fed. Proc. Fed. Am. Soc. Exp. Biol.,* 44, 134, 1985.
184. Castelli, W. P., Gordon, T., Hjortland, M. C., Kagan, A., Doyle, J. T., Hames, C. G., Hulley, S. B., and Zukel, W. J., Alcohol and blood lipids, *Lancet,* 2, 153, 1977.
185. Yano, K., Rhoads, G. G., and Kagan, A., Coffee, alcohol and risk of coronary heart disease among Japanese men living in Hawaii, *N. Engl. J. Med.,* 297, 405, 1977.
186. Sane, T., Nikkila, E. A., Taskinen, M., Valmaki, M., and Ylikahri, R., Accelerated turnover of very low density lipoprotein triglycerides in chronic alcohol users: a possible mechanism for the up-regulation of high density lipoprotein by ethanol, *Atherosclerosis,* 53, 185, 1984.
187. Cluette, J. E., Mulligan, J. J., Noring, R., Igoe, F. D., and Hojnacki, J. L., Effect of ethanol on lipoprotein synthesis and fecal sterol excretion, *Nutr. Res.,* 5, 45, 1985.
188. Eberhard, T. P., Effect of alcohol on cholesterol-induced atherosclerosis in rabbits, *Arch. Pathol.,* 21, 616, 1936.
189. Goto, Y., Kikuchi, H., Abe, K., Nagawashi, Y., Ohira, S., and Kudo, H., The effect of ethanol on the onset of experimental atherosclerosis, *Tohoku J. Exp. Med.,* 114, 35, 1974.
190. Klatsky, A. L., Friedman, G. D., and Sregelaub, A. B., Alcohol consumption before myocardial infarction: results from the Kaiser-Permanente epidemiologic study of myocardial infarction, *Ann. Intern. Med.,* 81, 294, 1974.
191. Kannel, B. and Gordon, T., Eds., The Framingham Study, Washington, D.C., Government Printing Office, Section 26, 1970.
192. Dyer, A. R., Stamler, J., Paul, O., Lepper, M., Shekelle, R. B., McKean, H., and Garside, D., Alcohol consumption and 17-year mortality in the Chicago Western Electric Company study, *Prev. Med.,* 9, 78, 1980.
193. Barboriak, J. J., Rimm, A. A., Anderson, A. J., Schmidhoffer, M., and Tristani, F. E., Coronary artery occlusion and alcohol intake, *Br. Heart J.,* 39, 289, 1977.
194. Colditz, G. A., Branch, L. G., Lipnick, R. J., Willet, W. C., Rosner, B., Posner, B., and Hennekens, C. H., Moderate alcohol and decreased cardiovascular mortality in an elderly cohort, *Am. Heart J.,* 109, 886, 1985.
195. Barboriak, J. J. and Menahan, L. A., Alcohol, lipoproteins and coronary heart disease, *Heart Lung,* 8, 736, 1979.
196. Segal, L. D., Klausner, S. C., Harney-Gnadt, J. T., and Amsterdam, E. A., Alcohol and the heart, *Med. Clin. N. Am.,* 68, 147, 1984.
197. Ehinger, P. O. and Regan, T. J., Does low-dose alcohol protect against coronary artery disease?, *J. Cardiol. Med.,* 5, 253, 1980.
198. Friedman, H. S., Alcohol and heart disease, *Primary Cardiol.,* 44, 1984.
199. Barboriak, J. J., Anderson, A. J., Rimm, A. A., and King, J. F., High density lipoprotein cholesterol and coronary artery occlusion, *Metabolism,* 28, 735, 1979.
200. Barboriak, J. J., Anderson, A. J., and Hoffmann, R. G., Interrelationship between coronary artery occlusion, high-density lipoprotein cholesterol, and alcohol intake, *J. Lab. Clin. Med.,* 94, 348, 1979.
201. Gruchow, H. W., Hoffman, R. G., Anderson, A. J., and Barboriak, J. J., Effects of drinking patterns on the relationship between alcohol and coronary occlusion, *Atherosclerosis,* 43, 393, 1982.
202. Barboriak, J. J., Gruchow, H. W., and Anderson, A. J., Pattern of alcohol intake and blood lipid levels, *Clin. Exp. Res.,* 6, 135, 1982.
203. Barboriak, J. J., Jacobson, G. R., Cushman, P., Herrington, R. E., Lipo, R. F., Daley, M. E., and Anderson, A. J., Chronic alcohol abuse and high density lipoprotein cholesterol, alcoholism, *Clin. Exp. Res.,* 4, 346, 1980.
204. Willet, W., Hennekens, C. H., Siegel, A. J., Adner, M. M., and Castelli, W. P., Alcohol consumption and high density lipoprotein cholesterol in marathon runners, *N. Engl. J. Med.,* 303, 1159, 1980.
205. Hartung, G. H., Foreyt, J. P., Mitchell, R. E., Mitchell, J. G., Reeves, R. S., and Gotto, A. M., Jr., Effect of alcohol intake on high-density lipoprotein cholesterol levels in runners and inactive men, *JAMA,* 249, 747, 1983.
206. Camargo, C. A., Williams, P. T., Vranizan, K. M., Albers, J. J., and Wood, P. D., The effect of moderate alcohol intake on serum apolipoproteins A-I and A-II, *JAMA,* 253, 2854, 1985.
207. LaPorte, R., Valvo-Gerard, L., Kuller, L., Dai, W., Bates, M., Cresanta, J., Williams, K., and Palkin, D., The relationship between alcohol consumption, liver enzymes and high-density lipoprotein cholesterol, *Circulation,* 64, 67, 1981.
208. Devenyi, P., Kapur, B. M., and Roy, J. H. J., High-density lipoprotein response to alcohol consumption and abstinence as an indicator of liver function in alcoholic patients, *Can. Med. Assoc. J.,* 130, 1445, 1984.
209. Avogaro, P., Cazzolato, G., Belussi, F., and Bittolo Bon, G., Altered apoprotein composition of HDL_2 and HDL_3 in chronic alcoholics, *Artery,* 10, 317, 1982.
210. Rosseneu, M., Stellemans, G., Vercaemst, R., and Belpairs, F., Plasma apoprotein levels in chronic alcohol abuse, *Artery,* 10, 193, 1982.

211. Nestel, P. J., Tada, N., and Fidge, N. H., Increased catabolism of high density lipoprotein in alcoholic hepatitis, *Metabolism,* 29, 101, 1980.
212. Okazaki, M., Hara, I., and Tanaka, A., Decreased serum HDL$_3$ cholesterol levels in cirrhosis of the liver, *N. Engl. J. Med.,* 304, 1608, 1981.
213. Gidez, L. I., Miller, G. J., Burstein, M., Slagle, S., and Eder, H. A., Separation and quantitation of subclasses of human plasma high density lipoproteins by a simple precipitation procedure, *J. Lipid Res.,* 23, 1206, 1982.
214. Morello, A. M. and Nicolosi, R. J., Electrophoretic profiles of high density lipoprotein subclasses in primates, *Comp. Biochem. Physiol.,* 69B, 291, 1981.
215. Rose, H. G. and Juliano, J., Regulation of plasma lecithin:cholesterol acyltransferase in man. III. Role of high density lipoprotein cholesteryl esters in the activating effect of a high-fat test meal, *J. Lipid Res.,* 20, 399, 1979.
216. Marx, J. L., The HDL: the good cholesterol carriers?, *Science,* 205, 677, 1979.
217. Lieber, C. S., To drink (moderately) or not to drink?, *N. Engl. J. Med.,* 310, 846, 1984.
218. Duhamel, G., Forgez, P., Nalpas, B., Berthelot, P., and Chapman, M. J., Spur cells in patients with alcoholic liver cirrhosis are associated with reduced plasma levels of apo A-II, HDL$_3$ and LDL, *J. Lipid Res.,* 24, 1612, 1983.
219. Haffner, S. M., Applebaum-Bowden, D., Wahl, P. W., Hoover, J. J., Warnick, G. R., Albers, J. J., and Hazzard, W. R., Epidemiological correlates of high denstiy lipoprotein subfractions, apolipoproteins A-I, A-II, and D, and lecithin cholesterol acyltransferase: effects of smoking, alcohol, and adiposity, *Arteriosclerosis,* 5, 169, 1985.
220. Williams, P. T., Krauss, R. M., Wood, P. D., Albers, J. J., Dreun, D., and Ellsworth, N., Associations of diet and alcohol intake with high-density lipoprotein subclasses, *Metabolism,* 34, 524, 1985.
221. Danielsson, B., Ekman, R., Fex, G., Johansson, B. G., Kristensson, H., Nilsson-Ehle, P., and Wadstein, J., Changes in plasma high density lipoproteins in chronic male alcoholics during and after abuse, *Scand. J. Clin. Lab. Invest.,* 38, 113, 1978.
222. Cluette, J. E., Mulligan, J. J., Noring, R., Doyle, K., and Hojnacki, J. L., Ethanol enhances *de novo* synthesis of high density lipoprotein cholesterol, *Proc. Soc. Exp. Biol. Med.,* 176, 508, 1984.
223. Paterniti, J. R., Brown, W. V., and Ginsbert, H. M., Combined lipase deficiency: a lethal mutation on chromosome 17 of the mouse, *Science,* 221, 167, 1982.
224. Mikkila, E. A., Taskinen, M., and Huttunen, J. K., Effect of acute ethanol load on postheparin plasma lipoprotein lipase and hepatic lipase activities and intravenous fat tolerance, *Horm. Metab. Res.,* 1978.
225. Karsenty, C., Baraona, E., Savolainen, M. J., and Lieber, C. S., Effects of chronic ethanol intake on mobilization and excretion of cholesterol in baboons, *J. Clin. Invest.,* 75, 976, 1985.
226. Lee, H., Noel, S. P., Hosein, E. A., and Rubenstein, D., Secretion of high density lipoprotein by the isolated perfused alcoholic rat liver, *Experientia,* 38, 914, 1982.
227. Jenkins, D. J. A., Dietary fibre, diabetes and hyperlipidemia, *Lancet,* 2, 1287, 1979.
228. Liebman, M., Smith, M. C., Iverson, J., Thye, F. W., Hinkle, D. E., et al., Effects of course wheat bran fiber and exercise on plasma lipids and lipoproteins in moderately overweight men, *Am. J. Clin. Nutr.,* 36, 71, 1983.
229. Kay, R. M., Sabry, Z. I., and Csima, A., Multivariate analysis of diet and serum lipids, *Am. J. Clin. Nutr.,* 33, 2566, 1980.
230. Raymond, T. L., Connor, W. E., Lin, D. S., Warner, S., Fry, M. M., and Connor, S. L., The interaction of dietary fibers and cholesterol upon the plasma lipids and lipoproteins, sterol balance and bowel function in human subjects, *J. Clin. Invest.,* 60, 1429, 1977.
231. Arvanitakis, C., Stammes, C. L., Folscroft, J., and Beyer, P., Failure of bran to alter diet-induced hyperlipidemia in the rat, *Proc. Soc. Exp. Biol. Med.,* 154, 550, 1977.
232. Munoz, J. M., Sandstead, H. H., Jacob, R. A., Logan, G. M., Reck, S. J., Klevay, L. M., Dintzis, F. R., Inglett, G. F., and Shuey, W. C., Effects of some cereal brans and textured vegetable protein on plasma lipids, *Am. J. Clin. Nutr.,* 32, 580, 1979.
233. Walters, R. L., McLean, I., Davies, P. S., Hill, M. J. K., Drasar, B. S., Southgate, D. A. T., and Morgan, B., Effects of two types of dietary fibre on fecal steroid and lipid excretion, *Br. Med. J.,* 2, 536, 1975.
234. Kretsch, M. J., Crawford, L. K., and Calloway, D. H., Some aspects of bile acid and urobilinogen excretion and fecal elimination in men given a rural Guatemalan diet and egg formulas with and without added oat bran, *Am. J. Clin. Nutr.,* 32, 1492, 1979.
235. Kirby, R. W., Anderson, J. W., Sieling, B., Rees, E. D., Chen, W. J. L., Miller, R. E., and Kay, R. M., Oat bran intake selectively lowers serum low density lipoprotein concentrations: studies of hypercholesterolemic men, *Am. J. Clin. Nutr.,* 34, 824, 1981.
236. Anderson, J. W., Kirby, R. W., and Rees, E. D., Oat bran selectively lowers serum low-density lipoprotein cholesterol concentrations in men, *Am. J. Clin. Nutr.,* 33, 914, 1980.

237. Kay, R. M. and Truswell, A. S., Effect of citrus pectin on blood lipids and fecal steroid excretion in man, *Am. J. Clin. Nutr.,* 30, 171, 1977.

238. Kay, R. M., Judd, P. A., and Truswell, A. S., The effect of pectin on serum cholesterol, *Am. J. Clin. Nutr.,* 31, 562, 1978.

239. Thiffault, C., Belander, M., and Pouliot, M., Traitement de l'hyperlipoproteinemie essentielle de type II par un nouvel agent therapeutique, la celluline, *Can. Med. Assoc. J.,* 103, 165, 1970.

240. Jenkins, D. J. A., Leeds, A. R., Slavin, B., Mann, J., and Jepson, E. M., Dietary fibre in blood lipids: reduction of serum cholesterol in type II hyperlipidemia by guargum, *Am. J. Clin. Nutr.,* 32, 16, 1979.

241. Jenkins, D. J. A., Reynolds, D., Slavin, B., Leeds, A. R., Jenkins, A. W., and Jepson, E. M., Dietary fiber and blood lipids: treatment of hypercholesterolemia with guar crispbread, *Am. J. Clin. Nutr.,* 33, 575, 1980.

242. Simons, L. A., Gayst, S., Balasubramaniam, S., and Ruys, J., Long-term treatment of hypercholesterolemia with a new palatable formulation of guargum, *Atherosclerosis,* 45, 101, 1982.

243. Miettinen, T. A. and Tarpila, S., Effects of pectin on serum cholesterol, fecal bile acids and biliary lipids in normolipidemic and hyperlipidemic individuals, *Clin. Chim. Acta,* 79, 471, 1977.

244. Kay-McPherson, R., Dietary fiber, *J. Lipid Res.,* 23, 221, 1982.

Chapter 7

USE OF DIET TO MODIFY SERUM CHOLESTEROL, LIPOPROTEINS, AND PROGRESSION OF CORONARY ATHEROSCLEROSIS

D. Kromhout and A. C. Arntzenius

TABLE OF CONTENTS

I. INTRODUCTION

In the U.S. remarkable changes in the food consumption pattern have taken place during the last 30 years. Total fat intake remained roughly the same with 40% of energy intake but the polyunsaturated-to-saturated fat ratio (P:S ratio) increased from 0.35 in the 1950s to 0.50 in the 1970s.[1] Also the cholesterol intake decreased during this period from 700 to 480 mg/day. The average serum total cholesterol level among U.S. middle-aged populations dropped during that period from 230 to 200 mg/dℓ. These changes were paralleled by a reduction in coronary heart disease (CHD) mortality of 2% per year since 1968.

In the Netherlands a change in P:S ratio was also observed between 1960 and 1980, namely from 0.33 to 0.57.[2] Dietary cholesterol consumption did not change but the fish and alcohol consumption increased during this period. There is evidence from population studies carried out in the Netherlands among males aged 40 to 49 that the average serum cholesterol level dropped by 14 mg/dℓ between 1960 and 1977 to 1978.[3,4] Since 1972 a 1.3% decrease per year is observed in CHD mortality among the Dutch population.[2]

These results suggest that on the population level, changes in fatty acid composition of the diet are followed by changes in serum total cholesterol and CHD mortality. These associations do not prove that the observed changes are causally related to each other but are consistent with the hypothesis that changes in the diet may modify serum total cholesterol levels and CHD mortality. Intervention studies are needed to provide definitive evidence for the diet-heart hypothesis. The results of dietary intervention on serum cholesterol, lipoproteins, CHD incidence and mortality, and progression of coronary atherosclerosis will be reviewed. Special attention will be paid to the results of the Leiden Intervention Trial.

II. EFFECT OF DIETARY INTERVENTION ON SERUM CHOLESTEROL AND LIPOPROTEINS

Intervention studies carried out in the 1950s and 1960s have shown that saturated fats elevate serum total cholesterol, monounsaturated fats are neutral, and polyunsaturated fats decrease serum total cholesterol.[5] Saturated fats are generally twice as effective in increasing serum total cholesterol than polyunsaturated fats in decreasing. Dietary cholesterol increases serum total cholesterol but its effect is smaller than that of saturated fats and is no longer present at a cholesterol intake of more than 800 mg/day.[6] The effect of changes in different fatty acids and dietary cholesterol on serum total cholesterol can be summarized in the Key's equation:[3]

$\Delta TC = 1.35 (2\Delta S - \Delta P) + 1.5 \Delta\sqrt{Z}$
TC = serum total cholesterol (mg/dℓ)
S = saturated fat (%E)
P = polyunsaturated fat (%E)
Z = dietary cholesterol (mg per 1000 kcal)

Large scale intervention studies have shown that changes in fatty acid and cholesterol composition of the diet are accompanied by changes in serum total cholesterol of 10 to 15%.[7] Besides fatty acids and dietary cholesterol other components of the diet influence lipids and lipoproteins. It is therefore of interest to see whether more comprehensive changes in the diet lead to larger changes in lipids and lipoproteins. Such an intervention study was done by Lewis and co-workers.[8] They compared a diet with

27% of energy from fat, P:S ratio 1.0, 100 mg dietary cholesterol per 1000 kcal, and 22 g dietary fiber per 1000 kcal with a Western reference diet, e.g., 40% of energy from fat, P:S ratio 0.27, 250 mg dietary cholesterol per 1000 kcal, and 8 g dietary fiber per 1000 kcal. The fat modified, dietary-fiber enriched diet reduced serum total cholesterol by 29.2%, LDL cholesterol by 34.5%, VLDL triglycerides by 19.0%, and HDL cholesterol by 10.6%.

Similar results were obtained in an intervention study carried out by Enholm and co-workers among middle-aged volunteers in North Karelia, Finland.[9] A change from their usual diet (total fat: 39% of energy, P:S ratio 0.2, and dietary cholesterol 185 mg per 1000 kcal) to a Mediterranean-type diet (total fat: 24% of energy, P:S ratio 1.2, and dietary cholesterol 125 mg per 1000 kcal) lead to significant changes in serum total cholesterol and lipoprotein concentrations. The average serum total cholesterol level dropped by 23.5% among males and 21.4% among females and HDL cholesterol by 18.5% among males and 16.1% among females.

The results of the intervention studies carried out by Lewis and co-workers and by Enholm and co-workers showed that substantial changes in serum total cholesterol and lipoproteins can be obtained by changing the fatty acid, dietary cholesterol, and dietary fiber content of the diet.[8,9] Besides a desired decrease in serum total cholesterol also a reduction in HDL cholesterol was observed in these intervention studies. HDL cholesterol is inversely related to CHD incidence.[10] In future intervention studies different diets should be tested with the aim to reduce serum total cholesterol as much as possible and not to reduce HDL cholesterol. A recently reported intervention study suggests that a diet high in monounsaturated fat is as effective as a diet high in polyunsaturated fat in lowering serum total cholesterol but does not reduce HDL cholesterol.[11]

III. SERUM TOTAL CHOLESTEROL AND CHD

Many clinical trials of serum total cholesterol lowering have been reported.[12] These trials have studied persons with and without clinical signs of CHD and have used diet or drugs. Conventionally coronary heart disease incidence and mortality are used as endpoints in these trials. The results of these trials suggest that serum total cholesterol lowering is associated with a reduction in CHD incidence and mortality but are inconclusive. Recently however, the Lipid Research Clinic Primary Prevention Trial has shown that lowering of serum total and LDL cholesterol by diet and cholestyramine was followed by a significant reduction in coronary heart disease incidence and mortality.[13,14] On average a reduction of serum total cholesterol by 1% was paralleled by a reduction of 2% in CHD incidence during 7.4 years of follow-up.

An alternative strategy to evaluate the efficacy of lipid lowering is to use the rate of change in arterial lesions as an endpoint. Nine of the latter type of studies have been published.[15-23] The results of these intervention studies published between 1975 and 1985 are summarized in Table 1. They were almost all small-scale studies with between 24 and 42 subjects except the NHLBI Type II Coronary Intervention Study with 116 subjects. The intervention period was generally relatively short, 1 to 3 years, again with the exception of the NHLBI Type II Study which lasted 5 years. Only 3 of the 9 studies included a control group. Changes in arterial lesions were measured on the angiograms. By one investigator this was done by a vernier caliper device, in five studies the angiograms were "read" by one or more experienced cardiologists by eye and in three studies the angiograms were "read" by eye as well as by computer processing. In 7 of the 9 trials changes in the arterial lesions were correlated with the serum total cholesterol levels of the participants. In 8 of the 9 trials intervention was done by drug treatment with or without diet. The Leiden Intervention Trial differed from the others

Table 1

INTERVENTION STUDIES USING ARTERIAL LESIONS AS ENDPOINT

Authors	Year	Number	Artery	Duration (years)	Drugs	Diet	Control group	Measurement techniques	Serum cholesterol and lesion change
Cohn, et al.	1975	40	Coronary	1	Clofibrate	–	+	Eye (4)[a]	–
Blankenhorn, et al.	1978	25	Femoral	1	Clofibrate Neomycin	+	–	Eye and computer	+
Rafflenbeul, et al.	1979	25	Coronary	1	Optimal treatment	–	–	Vernier caliper	–
Kuo, et al.	1979	25	Coronary	3	Colestipol	+	–	Eye (3)	+
Nash, et al.	1982	42	Coronary	2	Colestipol	–	–	Eye (2)	+
Duffield, et al.	1983	24	Femoral	1 1/2	Cholestyramine Nicotinic acid Clofibrate	+	+	Eye and computer	+
Nikkila, et al.	1983	30	Coronary	3	Clofibrate Nicotinic acid	+	–	Eye (2)	+
Levy, et al.	1984	116	Coronary	5	Cholestyramine	+	+	Eye (3)	+
Arntzenius, et al.	1985	39	Coronary	2	—	+	–	Eye (2) and computer	+

[a] ( ) Number of cardiologists.

because lipid lowering was obtained solely by dietary measures.[23] The results of this trial will be discussed in detail.

IV. THE LEIDEN INTERVENTION TRIAL

The trial was conducted between 1978 and 1982. Patients with stable angina pectoris in whom coronary arteriography had demonstrated severe narrowing of the diameter ($\geqslant 50\%$) of one of the major coronary arteries, were selected for the trial. Each patient followed a diet for 2 years, during which the usual, appropriate individual therapy was also given for angina pectoris, elevated blood pressure, cardiac arrhythmias, and symptoms of heart failure, e.g., beta-blockers, diuretics, digitalis, nitroglycerin, and anticoagulants. The participants were seen 15 times during the 2-year period by cardiologists and dieticians. Of the 53 patients who entered the study, 4 died during the first year, 3 of acute myocardial infarction and 1 suddenly. In 7 patients with two-vessel disease, the angina became labile and necessitated coronary bypass surgery. Repeat angiography was not carried out in 3 patients; malignant disease had developed in 2, and the second investigtion was refused by one. Complete information was available for 39 patients. The 35 men and 4 women were between 33 and 59 years of age with an average of 48.9.

A. Diet

Intervention consisted of a linoleic acid-enriched diet with a P:S ratio of 2 and a dietary cholesterol intake of less than 100 mg/day. This was obtained by using polyunsaturated fat rich oils and margarines and by exchanging meat and meat products with specially prepared vegetable protein rich substitutes (details on the composition of the baseline and intervention diet are given in the appendix). Much emphasis was placed on continuous supervision and dietary instruction for the patients and their spouses. Instruction was individualized and based on 24-hour recall of food intake, which was recorded before intervention. To evaluate adherence one year after the trial had begun information on food intake was collected by 7-day record under supervision of a dietician.

Dietary information at baseline and after 1 year of intervention was collected at 28 of the 39 patients. It is unlikely that these 28 patients represented biased selection from among the 39, because at baseline the food intake of the 28 did not differ significantly from that of the 10 patients who participated in the baseline survey only. All foods and drinks were coded and analyzed according to the Uniform Food Encoding System, developed in the Netherlands. For the present analyses the extended computerized version of the Netherlands Food Table from 1984 was used. The fatty acid composition of foods in this version of the food table was more complete than in earlier versions. The results presented in this chapter may therefore differ somewhat from those presented earlier.[23]

At baseline the diet contained an average of 1988 kcal/day, had a P:S ratio of 0.73 and had a cholesterol content of 97.8 mg per 1000 kcal (Table 2). In the Dutch population in general the P:S ratio is 0.57 and dietary cholesterol is 140 mg per 1000 kcal.[2] These data suggest that the participating patients were already following some type of a cholesterol-lowering diet before they entered the study. They were then placed on the linoleic acid-enriched diet with a P:S ratio of 2 and a dietary cholesterol intake of less than 100 mg/day. Compliance was measured by dietary surveys and by analyses of the serum linoleic acid content of the cholesteryl esters. The surveys showed that after 1 year of intervention the average P:S ratio was 1.92 and the average dietary cholesterol intake 28.8 mg per 1000 kcal (Table 2). These results indicate that the patients reduced

Table 2

ENERGY AND MACRONUTRIENTS AT BASELINE
AND AFTER 1 YEAR OF INTERVENTION IN 28 OF
THE 39 PATIENTS

Dietary variable		Baseline m ± s.d.	One year m ± s.d.
Energy	(kcal)	1988 ± 522	1946 ± 571
Vegetable protein	(%E)	5.1 ± 1.2	6.9 ± 1.4[a]
Animal protein	(%E)	11.6 ± 3.4	8.0 ± 3.7[a]
Total protein	(%E)	16.6 ± 3.6	14.8 ± 3.4
Saturated fat	(%E)	13.6 ± 4.8	9.1 ± 2.1[a]
Monounsaturated fat	(%E)	11.4 ± 4.6	6.9 ± 1.6[a]
Polyunsaturated fat	(%E)	8.8 ± 3.5	17.2 ± 5.0[a]
P:S ratio[b]	(%E)	0.73 ± 0.40	1.92 ± 0.50[a]
Total fat	(%E)	34.3 ± 8.7	33.6 ± 7.7
Dietary cholesterol	(mg/mcal)	97.8 ± 32.4	28.8 ± 20.1[a]
Oligosaccharides	(%E)	22.0 ± 6.4	21.8 ± 5.3
Polysaccharides	(%E)	23.4 ± 4.9	26.5 ± 5.7[c]
Total carbohydrates	(%E)	45.5 ± 7.4	48.5 ± 6.4
Alcohol	(%E)	3.5 ± 5.5	3.1 ± 4.1
Dietary fiber	(g/mcal)	13.3 ± 4.8	16.3 ± 4.4[c]

[a] $p \leqslant 0.001$

[b] $p \leqslant 0.05$

[c]   P:S ratio denotes ratio of polyunsaturated to saturated fat.

their intake of saturated fat by about 35% and doubled their intake of polyunsaturated fat. The latter finding was confirmed by a significant increase from 52.4 to 60.8% in the linoleic acid content of the serum cholesteryl esters. On the basis of changes in the fatty acid and cholesterol content of the diet, the expected decrease in average serum total cholesterol level could be calculated according to Keys' equation.[5] The expected decrease did not differ from the observed (−0.78 vs. −0.82 mmol/l [−30.2 vs. −31.7 mg/dl]).

Besides the changes in P:S ratio and dietary cholesterol the intervention diet contained more vegetable protein, polysaccharides, and dietary fiber due to a higher intake of cereals, vegetarian meat substitutes, raw vegetables, and fruits, compared with the baseline diet (Table 2, Appendix). During the intervention period body weight, Quetelet Index, serum total cholesterol, total/HDL cholesterol, and systolic blood pressure dropped significantly (Table 3). The 3% decrease in HDL cholesterol was not statistically significant. In the intervention studies reported by Lewis and Enholm a significant decrease in HDL cholesterol was observed.[8,9] The diets of all three intervention studies were characterized by P:S ratios of between one and two. There was, however, a difference in total fat intake. This amounted to 34% of total energy in the Leiden study and to, respectively, 27 and 24% of total energy in the two other studies.[8,9] Lewis, in addition, studied the effect of a diet with a P:S ratio of 1.0 and a total fat intake of 40% of total energy and found, consistent with the Leiden findings, a nonsignificant decrease of 5.5% in HDL cholesterol.[9] It may be concluded that besides the fatty acid composition also the total amount of fat is of importance in relation to HDL cholesterol levels.

B. Coronary Artery Lesions

Coronary arteriography has been performed in all patients immediately before entry. The initial visual assessment of the angiograms was conducted by a clinical angiogra-

Table 3

CHANGES IN VALUES FOR RISK FACTORS IN THE 39 PATIENTS OVER 2 YEARS[a]

Risk factors		At baseline	At 2 years	Change
Body weight	(kg)	74.5 ± 11.4	73.5 ± 11.3	−1.2 ± 3.6[b]
Quetelet Index	(kg/m²)	24.0 ± 2.4	23.7 ± 2.6	−0.4 ± 1.1[b]
Serum total cholesterol	(mmol/ℓ)[c]	6.9 ± 1.4	6.2 ± 1.3	−0.7 ± 0.7[d]
HDL cholesterol	(mmol/ℓ)[c]	1.01 ± 0.21	0.98 ± 0.16	−0.03 ± 0.14
Total/HDL cholesterol		7.1 ± 1.8	6.4 ± 1.6	−0.6 ± 1.2[e]
Systolic blood pressure	(mmHg)	130.4 ± 17.4	126.3 ± 14.2	−4.2 ± 11.2[b]
Diastolic blood pressure	(mmHg)	84.4 ± 11.1	82.1 ± 7.6	−2.4 ± 8.5
Smoking	(No. of patients)	18	18[f]	0

[a]   Values are means ± s.d.
[b]   Significant difference ($p < 0.05$).
[c]   To convert to milligrams per deciliter, multiply by 38.7.
[d]   Significant difference ($p < 0.001$).
[e]   Significant difference ($p < 0.01$).
[f]   Includes four patients who stopped smoking during the second year of intervention.

pher. Patients with at least one obstruction of 50% or more were invited to enroll in the study. The examination was repeated, as scheduled, after 2 years of dietary intervention.

Films were assessed visually by two experienced observers who had no knowledge of the lipid values and who could not distinguish between the first and second angiograms since identical techniques had been used and since the dates of the films were concealed.

Computer-assisted analysis was carried out with the computer-based Coronary Angiography Analysis System (CAAS, Thorax Center, Rotterdam). This system permits the accurate delineation of the contours of user-selected coronary arterial segments by means of automated edge-detection algorithms.

In order to evaluate the variability of the measurements, end-diastolic cine frames of 13 routine coronary angiograms were analyzed twice by one technician, with a median interval of 28 days between analyses. The average difference between duplicate measurements was found to be 0.00 mm; the variability, defined as the standard deviation of the differences between repeated measurements, was found to be 0.10 mm.[24] According to computer assessment, a total of 166 lesions (of which the least stenosis measured 0.14 mm) were detected in the 11 major epicardial coronary segments. On average, the patients had 4.26 ± 1.52 lesions. Seven patients had one-vessel disease, 11 had two-vessel disease, and 21 had three-vessel disease.

The mean diameter of vessels at the 166 sites of obstruction was 2.12 ± 0.99 mm on the first arteriogram and 1.99 ± 1.01 mm on the second, illustrating that on average, the coronary lesions of the 39 patients progressed during 2 years of observation ($p < 0.01$). Similar results were found using visual assessment of the lesions. Progression of lesions was defined as a decrease of 0.1 mm or more in the mean coronary diameter (computer assessment) or as an increase in the mean percentage of narrowing (visual assessment). Both visual and computer-assisted assessment showed progression in 21 of the 39 patients but no lesion growth in 18 patients.

C. Total/HDL Cholesterol and Coronary Lesions

Computer-measured lesion growth correlated positively with the mean of the values for total/HDL cholesterol during 2 years of intervention (r = 0.39, p = 0.01). Stronger

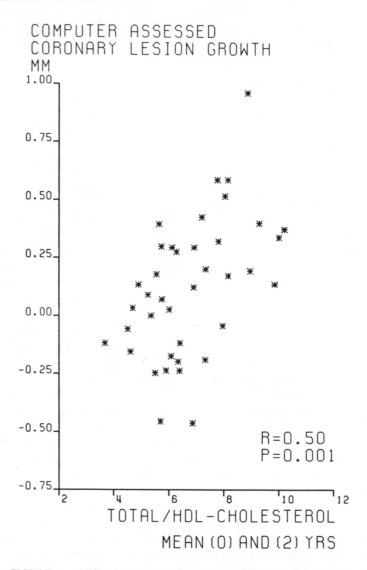

FIGURE 1.   Association between change in coronary lesion and the ratio
of total to high-density-lipoprotein (total/HDL) cholesterol according to individual patient. Values for total/HDL cholesterol are averages of baseline
and mean 2-year values for 39 patients. Progression of lesion growth (values
above 0.1 mm) is associated with relatively high values for total/HDL cholesterol. Mainly, patients with relatively low values for total/HDL cholesterol had no disease progression — some men had regression.

associations were found with the baseline total/HDL cholesterol ($r = 0.55$, $p < 0.001$)
and the average of baseline and 2 years intervention ($r = 0.50$, $p = 0.001$) (Figure 1).
The stronger association for the baseline total/HDL cholesterol values may be due to
a larger range in the baseline values (95% of the values between 3.46 and 10.68) than
in the values during intervention (3.32 and 9.56), since all patients were put on the
same diet. A strong correlation was observed between total/HDL cholesterol at baseline and during 2 years of intervention ($r = 0.78$, $p < 0.001$). We therefore conclude
that in the Leiden Intervention Trial coronary lesion growth was strongly related to
total/HDL cholesterol. In six of the eight intervention studies reported also associations were found between serum total cholesterol levels and the likelihood of progres-

sion of coronary atherosclerotic lesion growth as assessed by repeat arteriography (Table 1).

D. Diet, Total/HDL Cholesterol, and Coronary Lesion Growth

Because there was no control group, the effect of dietary intervention on total/HDL cholesterol level and coronary lesion growth could not be assessed directly. To obtain indirect information on the effect of the diet, data were stratified to total/HDL cholesterol level. The 19 patients with total/HDL cholesterol levels below the median (<6.9) were called "low" and the 20 patients with values above the median (>6.9) were called "high". Over the ensuing 2 years no change in the mean coronary diameter of the 19 low patients was observed (mean change, +0.002 mm), but a significant progression of the disease was found among the 20 high patients (mean change, −0.237 mm).

The 20 high patients were divided in two subgroups: the "high-high" subgroup, 11 patients whose total/HDL cholesterol remained above 6.9 during 2 years of intervention and the "high-low" subgroup, 9 patients whose ratio became below 6.9 during the 2 years of intervention. No progression of coronary lesions (mean change, −0.043 mm) was observed in the 9 high-low patients but the coronary lesions progressed significantly among the 11 high-high patients (mean change, −0.396 mm; $p = 0.01$) (Figure 2).

The fatty acid and cholesterol content of the diet was expressed as the so-called ϕ value, based on Keys' equation; $\phi = 1.35 (2S - P) + 1.5$ Z, where S denotes saturated fatty acids (percent energy), P, polyunsaturated fatty acids (percent energy), and Z, dietary cholesterol (milligrams per 1000 kcal) (Figure 2).[5] The values for saturated fatty acids and cholesterol content elevate the ϕ value, whereas the value for polyunsaturated fatty acids does the opposite. At baseline in the present study the highest ϕ value (52.2) as found among the high-low patients; it was similar to that of the Dutch population (47).[2] The baseline ϕ values of the low group and the high-high subgroup were lower (36.6 and 32.1, respectively). After 1 year of intervention, no differences between the ϕ values of the three groups were observed. The changes in the ϕ value (resulting from a lower saturated fat and cholesterol intake) was largest in the persons in the high-low group ($p < 0.05$). These patients showed in contrast to the high-high patients no progression of coronary lesions. These findings suggest that in patients with high values for total/HDL cholesterol and high ϕ values (e.g., similar to values in the general population of industrialized Western countries) dietary intervention may reduce the rate of coronary lesion growth.

V. CONCLUSIONS

Almost all intervention studies using coronary arteriography as an endpoint show that serum total cholesterol is related to coronary atherosclerotic lesion growth (Table 1). The only intervention study that used solely diet as mode of intervention suggests that dietary intervention may reduce the rate of coronary lesion growth.[23] The evidence provided by the intervention studies carried out until this moment is limited due to weaknesses in design, e.g., small number of subjects, short duration, no control group, etc. Larger controlled studies are needed to show that dietary intervention is effective in preventing coronary lesion growth. The results from different types of intervention studies carried out until this moment provide evidence that the total/HDL cholesterol ratio can be influenced by changing from high saturated fat — high cholesterol diet to a Mediterranean-type diet. This change will probably also be associated with a reduction in coronary lesion growth and in CHD incidence.

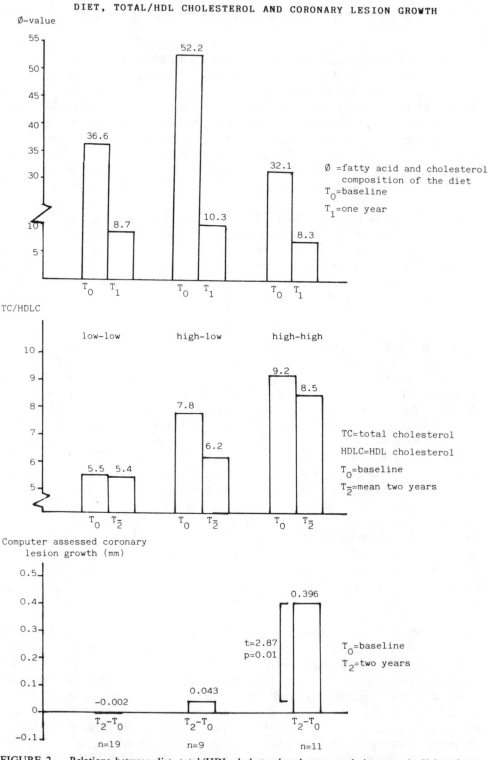

FIGURE 2.   Relations between diet, total/HDL cholesterol and coronary lesion growth. Values for ø (content of fatty acids and cholesterol in the diet, based on Keys' equation) are presented according to group. The low-low group had low levels (<6.9) for total/HDL cholesterol at baseline and during dietary intervention. The high-low group had high levels (>6.9) before and low levels (<6.9) during intervention. The high-high group had high levels (>6.9) before and during intervention. Disease progression occurred in the high-high group but not in the low-low and high-low group.

ACKNOWLEDGMENT

We are much indebted to N. Kempen-Voogd, dietician and J. W. van Wingen, programmer, for their help with the collection and analyses of the dietary data.

APPENDIX

Food Consumption Pattern (g/day) of 28 Patients with Stable Angina Pectoris
at Baseline and at 1 Year of Intervention

Food group	Baseline		One year	
	m	Range	m	Range
Bread (low fiber, <4 g/100 g)	18.6	0—154	6.9	0—35
Bread (high fiber, >4 g/100 g)	124.1	0—309	142.3	30—329
Cereals (low fiber, <5 g/100 g)	15.5	0—269	33.9	0—110
Cereals (high fiber, >5 g/100 g)	2.8	0—43	10.0	0—101
Potatoes	151.5	0—343	124.0	9—288
Pulses	0.6	0—16	27.8	0—106
Vegetables prepared	191.4	50—400	190.8	87—466
Vegetables raw	4.9	0—60	60.0	0—333
Citrus fruits	32.2	0—223	33.0	0—174
Hard fruit, e.g., apples	113.6	0—334	132.9	0—334
Soft fruit, e.g., strawberries	—	—	19.8	0—130
Fruit preserves	8.7	0—86	16.7	0—74
Fruit juices	75.5	0—714	68.5	0—343
Peanuts	9.6	0—179	2.1	0—17
Nuts mixed	0.1	0—2	1.1	0—13
Sugar	26.8	0—84	15.6	0—71
Soft drinks	67.1	0—679	29.9	0—207
Chocolate	2.3	0—28	0.9	0—15
Licorice	—	—	0.8	0—13
Other sweets	15.0	0—77	19.9	0—102
Cookies and cakes	46.0	0—140	30.2	0—86
Hearty snacks	1.1	0—11	0.3	0—8
Beer	34.2	0—360	30.9	0—429
Wine	2.6	0—60	15.1	0—227
Other light alcoholic drinks	7.8	0—150	4.3	0—64
Spirits	21.5	0—111	19.3	0—129
Oils	0.1	0—3	4.4	0—17
Margarines (<40% PUFA)	8.1	0—30	—	—
Margarines (>40% PUFA)	17.6	0—51	46.7	2—119
Low fat margarines	2.3	0—31	0.1	0—4
Butter	0.5	0—14	—	—
Cooking fats	8.0	0—30	11.3	0—46
Milk products (≥8% fat)	8.7	0—60	31.2	0—124
Milk products (3—5% fat)	59.6	0—370	8.2	0—143
Milk products (<2% fat)	232.4	0—896	351.0	80—969
Eggs	3.2	0—15	9.7	0—43
Cheese (>15% fat)	28.1	0—111	—	—
Cheese (<15% fat)	16.8	0—104	47.2	9—140
Organ meat	—	—	0.8	0—18
Fat meat (>10% fat)	38.6	0—279	0.6	0—17
Lean meat (≤10% fat)	81.4	0—275	4.8	0—124
Meatproducts	23.2	0—99	0.2	0—6
Lean fish (≤5% fat)	4.3	0—43	23.3	0—52
Fatty fish (>5% fat)	0.6	0—17	—	—
Fish preserves	0.6	0—16	—	—
Seasonings	—	—	0.9	0—9

APPENDIX (continued)

Soups, sauces, dishes	0.5	0—14	28.4	0—82
Mineral water	37.2	0—200	28.0	0—157
Vegetarian meat substitutes	—	—	62.7	0—653

REFERENCES

1. Bierman, E. L., Does diet influence risk factors for cardiovascular disease?, Paper presented at the American Heart Association 57th Scientific Sessions, Miami Beach, Fla., November 12, 1984.
2. Kromhout, D. and Van Oostrom, M., Diet-heart hypotheses tested on the population level in the Netherlands between 1950 and 1980, in preparation, 1987.
3. Keys, A., *Seven Countries: A Multivariate Analyses of Death and Coronary Heart Disease,* Harvard University Press, Cambridge, Mass., 1980, 353.
4. Van Ree, J. W., Het Nijmeegs Interventie Project, Nijmegen, 1981.
5. Keys, A., Anderson, J. T., and Grande, F., Serum cholesterol response to changes in the diet. IV. Particular fatty acids in the diet, *Metabolism,* 14, 776, 1965.
6. Stamler, J., Diet, in *Ischaemic Heart Disease. The Strategy of Postponement,* Tybjaerg Hansen, A., Schnohr, P., and Rose, G., Eds., Year Book Medical Publishers, Chicago, 1977, 132.
7. Rifkind, B. M., Goor, R., and Schucker, B., Compliance and cholesterol-lowering in clinical trials: efficacy of diet, in *Atherosclerosis VI,* Schettler, G., Gotto, A. M., Middelhoff, G., Habenicht, A. J. R., and Jurutka, K. R., Eds., Springer Verlag, Berlin, 1983, 306.
8. Lewis, B., Hammett, F., Katan, M., Kay, R. M., Merkx, I., Nobels, A., Miller, N. E., and Swan, A. V., Toward an improved lipid-lowering diet: additive effects of changes in nutritent intake, *Lancet,* 2, 1310, 1981.
9. Enholm, C., Huttunen, J. K., Pietinen, P., Leino, U., Mutanen, M., Kostiainen, E., Pikkarainen, J., Dougherty, R., Iacono, J., and Puska, P., Effect of diet on serum lipoproteins in a population with a high risk of coronary heart disease, *N. Engl. J. Med.,* 307, 850, 1982.
10. Gordon, T., Castelli, W. P., Hjortland, M. C., Kannel, W. B., and Dawber, T. R., High density lipoprotein as a protective factor against coronary heart disease, *Am. J. Med.,* 62, 707, 1977.
11. Mattson, F. H. and Grundy, S. M., Comparison of effects of dietary saturated, monounsaturated, and polyunsaturated fatty acids on plasma lipid and lipoproteins, *J. Lipid Res.,* 26, 194, 1985.
12. Buchwald, H., Fitch, L., and Moore, R. B., Overview of randomized clinical trials of lipid intervention for atherosclerotic cardiovascular disease, *Controlled Clin. Trials,* 3, 271, 1982.
13. Lipid Research Clinics Program, The lipid research clinics coronary primary prevention trial results. I. Reduction in incidence of coronary heart disease, *JAMA,* 251, 351, 1984.
14. Lipid Research Clinics Program, The lipid research clinics coronary primary prevention trial results. II. The relationship of reduction in incidence of coronary heart disease to cholesterol lowering, *JAMA,* 251, 365, 1984.
15. Cohn, K., Sakai, F. J., and Langston, M. F., Jr., Effect of clofibrate on progression of coronary disease: a prospective angiographic study in man, *Am. Heart J.,* 89, 591, 1975.
16. Blankenhorn, D. H., Brooks, S. H., Selzer, R. H., and Barndt, R., Jr., The rate of atherosclerosis change during treatment of hyperlipoproteinemia, *Circulation,* 57, 355, 1978.
17. Rafflenbeul, W., Smith, L. R., Rogers, W. J., Mantle, J. A., Rackley, C. E., and Russell, R. O., Jr., Quantitative coronary arteriography: coronary anatomy of patients with unstable angina pectoris reexamined 1 year after optimal therapy, *Am. J. Cardiol.,* 43, 699, 1979.
18. Kuo, P. T., Hayase, K., Kostis, J. B., and Moreyra, A. E., Use of combined diet and colestipol in long-term (7 to 7 1/2 years) treatment of patients with type II hyperlipoproteinemia, *Circulation,* 59, 199, 1979.
19. Nash, D. T., Gensini, G., and Esente, P., Effect of lipid-lowering therapy on the progression of coronary atherosclerosis assessed by scheduled repetitive coronary arteriography, *Int. J. Cardiol.,* 2, 43, 1982.
20. Duffield, R. G. M., Lewis, B., Miller, N. E., Jamieson, C. W., Brunt, J. N. H., and Colchester, A. C. F., Treatment of hyperlipidaemia retards progression of symptomatic femoral atherosclerosis: a randomised controlled trial, *Lancet,* 2, 639, 1983.
21. Nikkilä, E. A., Viikinkoski, P., and Valle, M., Effect of lipid lowering treatment on progression of coronary atherosclerosis: a 7-year prospective angiographic study, *Circulation,* 68(Suppl. 3), 188, 1983.

22. Levy, R. I., Brensike, J. F., Epstein, S. E., Kelsey, S. F., Passamani, E. R., Richardson, J. M., Loh, I. K., Stone, N. J., Aldrich, R. F., Battaglini, J. W., Moriarty, D. J., and Detre, K. M., The influence of changes in lipid values induced by cholestyramine and diet on progression of coronary artery disease: results of the NHLBI Type II Coronary Intervention Study, *Circulation,* 69, 325, 1984.

23. Arntzenius, A. C., Kromhout, D., Barth, J. D., Reiber, J. H. C., Bruschke, A. V. G., Buis, B., Van Gent, C. M., Kempen-Voogd, N., Strikwerda, S., and Van der Velde, E. A., Diet, lipoproteins, and progression of coronary atherosclerosis. The Leiden intervention trial, *N. Engl. J. Med.,* 312, 805, 1985.

24. Reiber, J. H. C., Serruys, P. W., Kooyman, C. J., Wijns, W., Slager, C. J., Gerbrands, J. J., Schuurbiers, J. C. H., Den Boer, A., and Hugenholtz, P. G., Assessment of short-, medium-, and long-term variations in arterial dimensions from computer-assisted quantitation of coronary angiograms, *Circulation,* 71, 280, 1985.

Chapter 8

DIETARY INFLUENCE ON HYPERTENSION AND STROKE

Martina A. Diolulu

Increased peripheral vascular resistance is a common hemodynamic characteristic of spontaneously hypertensive rats (SHR),[1] and patients with essential hypertension.[2] The increased peripheral resistance is induced initially by neurogenic mechanisms as indicated by augmented sympathetic discharge,[3] increased norepinephrine turnover,[4] and increased serum dopamine-β-hydroxylase activity.[5] These neurogenic factors of hypertension are soon replaced by nonneurogenic mechanisms such as morphological alterations in the vessels as induced by accelerated protein synthesis,[6,7] and biochemical alterations in smooth muscle membranes of small resistance vessels,[8,9] and in sarcoplasmic reticulum (SR) function.[10,12] While the severity of neurogenically mediated hypertension can be reduced by chemical, pharmacological, or immunological manipulation,[13-15] recent findings indicate that it can also be influenced by dietary factors. Long-term feeding of a high protein diet maintains the elasticity and morphology of arterial walls in "stroke-prone" spontaneously hypertensive rats (SHRSP).[16] When SHRSP are fed a high protein diet, the urinary excretion of sodium is accelerated thus counteracting the adverse effect of salt on hypertension.[17] Dietary taurine[18] and methionine but not cysteine[16] markedly reduce blood pressure (BP) and the incidence of stroke in SHRSP; the results suggest a direct linkage between the sulfoamino acids and neural regulation of BP.

The possibility that the etiology of essential hypertension could be multifactorial has been discussed at length by Page.[19] Hypertension may also be due to hypercontractility of the vascular musculature. The final trigger for the contraction of all muscle is an increase in the concentration of cytosolic calcium. This concentration is controlled in most part by the activity of the sarcoplasmic reticulum pump which sequesters calcium during muscle relaxation and releases calcium during muscle contraction.[12,20] This hypothesis is of particular interest because Wei,[10] Bohr,[21] and Postnov et al.[22] demonstrated reduced ATP-dependent Ca^{2+}-transport activity of the sarcoplasmic reticulum isolated from SHR. These investigators suggested that such an alteration in Ca^{2+} transport could initiate a mechanism for maintaining high BP, one of the primary risk factors associated with the development of stroke in man.[23]

The effect of dietary factors on BP and the incidence of stroke as noted above led us to a study of the effects of diet on some biochemical parameters associated with myocardial Ca^{2+}-pump function.

Standard American rat food containing approximately 24% crude protein with 0.4% methionine (STD-diet) described by Knapka et al.[24] was modified[25] to provide two additional diets used in the current experiments (Tables 1 and 2). For a high protein diet (HP-diet), fish and soybean meal were substituted for corn and wheat grains thus increasing the content of crude protein to 32% with 0.7% methionine. For the third diet (MET-diet), 1.5% of the corn in the STD-diet was replaced with 1.5% methionine thus raising the content of methionine to 1.9% of the diet. A diet made to the formulation of the Funashahi-SP contained approximately 19% crude protein with 0.4% methionine,[26] and served as the low protein diet (LP-diet). All diets contained similar amounts of lipids with insignificant differences in vitamin and mineral content. The diets were purchased from a commercial manufacturer (Ziegler Brothers, Inc., Gardners, Pa.) in pellet form.

Table 1

COMPARISON OF THE FOUR LABORATORY STOCK DIETS

Nutrient	Japanese diet [J] (Funahashi-SP)	American diet [A] (NIH)	Methionine diet (MET-diet)	32% Protein (HP-diet)
Crude protein (%)	19.7	25.3	26.8	32.2
Crude fat (%)	4.8	5.3	4.8	4.1
Crude fiber (%)	3.4	3.5	3.4	4.0
Ash (%)	6.2	6.6	6.2	6.6
Minerals				
Calcium (%)	1.20	1.10	1.10	1.23
Phosphorus (%)	0.96	0.94	0.94	.97
Cobalt (ppm)	0.36	0.40	0.40	.76
Copper (ppm)	16.2	16.1	16.1	16.6
Iron (ppm)	214.0	255.0	255.0	359.0
Manganese (ppm)	52.6	61.1	61.1	103.0
Manganese (%)	0.26	0.19	0.19	.20
Zinc (ppm)	56.1	52.3	52.3	62.6
Iodine (ppm)	1.7	1.9	1.9	1.8
Selenium (ppm)	0.37	0.33	0.33	0.2
Vitamins				
Choline (%)	0.24	0.24	0.24	0.24
Niacin (ppm)	110.0	110.0	110.0	84.0
Pantothenic acid (ppm)	38.1	30.9	30.9	32.0
Pyridoxine (ppm)	12.0	10.0	10.0	15.4
Riboflavin (ppm)	10.0	8.0	8.0	10.5
Thiamine (ppm)	13.0	15.0	15.0	16.5
α-Tocopherol (ppm)	70.0	35.0	35.0	33.0

Note: The basic nutrient composition of the rat food was analyzed in multiple samples of each diet both in the U.S. and Japan. These analyses were performed by Lancaster Laboratories (Lancaster, Pennsylvania) in the U.S. and by Japan Food Research Laboratories (Tokyo) in Japan. While individual batches of diet can vary significantly in one or more components, the data reported here are the means of several analyses and representative of the most consistent composition. (From Yamori et al., *Hypertension,* 6, 49, 1984. With permission of American Heart Association.)

Animals were divided into four groups, housed under NIH standard animal housing conditions (constant temperature, humidity, and lighting), and maintained with free access to water and their respective experimental diet for 9 months.

The mean BP of rats on HP (225 mmHg) and MET (203 mmHg) were significantly lower ($p < 0.001$) than that of rats on LP (252 mmHg) and STD (247 mmHg) diets while the body weights were the same for all diet groups (Table 3). In an earlier study, Yamori et al. had shown that cerebral lesions occur in 88% of SHRSP on LP diet compared to 30% on STD diet (see Reference 26).

The animals were sacrificed at the age of 10 months and crude SR was isolated from their finely chopped and homogenized cardiac ventricles. SR was isolated via a modification of the method of Harigaya and Schwartz[27] as described in detail previously.[25] $(Ca^{2+}-Mg^{2+})$-ATPase, basal Mg^{2+}-ATPase as well as Ca^{2+} binding and uptake activities of the isolated SR were determined.

$Ca^{2+}-Mg^{2+}$-ATPase complexed with phospholipids forms an essential part of the active Ca^{2+}-transport system in the SR. The activity of this enzyme translocates Ca^{2+} into the interior of the SR.[12] This enzyme constitutes 60 to 80% of the total protein content

Table 2

ESSENTIAL AMINO ACID ANALYSIS OF HYDROLYZED RAT DIETS

Essential amino acid	Japanese Funahashi-SP diet [J] (mg/g)		American NIH diet [A] (mg/g)		Ratio A/J
	Mean	±SD	Mean	±SD	
Threonine	6.71	0.57	9.90	0.43	1.5
Valine	8.14	0.58	11.07	0.52	1.4
Methionine	2.76	0.38	4.57	0.15	1.7
Isoleucine	6.75	0.59	9.60	0.38	1.4
Leucine	12.53	1.41	19.50	1.03	1.6
Phenylalanine	7.43	1.03	10.43	0.57	1.4
Lysine	7.74	1.08	11.78	0.45	1.5
Histidine	5.83	1.55	5.65	0.94	1.0
Arginine	9.09	1.29	12.32	0.67	1.4
Total	66.95		94.82		1.4

Note: Values are means of five samples of different lots and denote significant differences from the Japanese diet.

[a] $p < 0.001$.

Adapted from Yamori, et al., *Hypertension*, 6, 49, 1984. With permission of American Heart Association.

Table 3

EFFECT OF DIET ON BLOOD PRESSURE (BP) AND BODY WEIGHT OF STROKE-PRONE RATS

	LP diet (n = 10)	STD diet (n = 10)	HP diet (n = 10)	MET diet (n = 10)
Body weight (g)	406 ± 4	404 ± 4	410 ± 3	414 ± 6
BP (mmHg)	252 ± 3	247 ± 3	225 ± 1[a]	203 ± 2[b]

Note: At 10 months of age the BP of each rat was measured by a tail cuff plethysmographic technique and body weights were recorded. (From Diolulu, M. A., et al., Clin. Exp. Hypertension, Theory and Practice: A 7(9), 1301, 1985. With permission.)

[a]   Significant difference from HP diet vs STD and LP diet group ($p < 0.001$).
[b]   Significant difference from MET diet vs STD and LP diet group ($p < 0.001$).

of SR and is important for the Ca^{2+} regulatory activity of the SR.[12,28] Comparison of data by analysis of variance and student's *t*-test indicates that the activity of (Ca^{2+}-Mg^{2+})-ATPase at all time periods was significantly higher in the SR fractions from SHRSP on MET-diet than that from the other diet groups (see Figure 1 and legend). By contrast, there were no significant changes in basal Mg^{2+}-ATPase activity in SR from SHRSP under the various experimental diets (data not shown).

Calcium binding was determined as described in detail previously.[25] The SR from all diet groups demonstrated time-dependent Ca^{2+} binding (Figure 2) that reached a steady

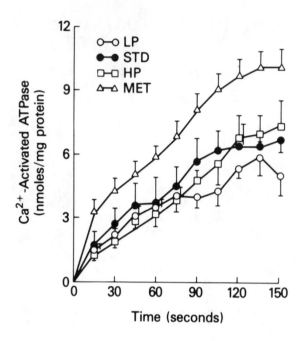

FIGURE 1.   Time course of $(Mg^{2+} + Ca^{2+})$-ATPase Activity in SR from SHRSP. Enzyme activity (P_i liberated) was determined as described in Materials and Methods.[20] Experimental data was compared by analysis of variance followed by student's *t*-test. Each data point represents the mean ± sem of five experiments using separate membrane preparations. MET vs. HP = $p < 0.01$ at 15 sec, $p < 0.001$ at 45 sec, $p < 0.005$ at 75 sec, $p < 0.025$ at 105 sec; MET vs. LP = $p < 0.025$ at 15 sec, $p < 0.005$ at 45 sec, $p < 0.025$ at 45 sec, $p < 0.001$ at 105 sec, $p < 0.005$ at 150 sec; MET vs STD = $p < 0.025$ at 150 sec. No other significant differences at these times. Statistical analyses were not computed for other time points. LP = low protein diet, STD = standard diet, HP = high protein diet, and MET = high methionine diet. (Diolulu, M. A., et al., *Clin. Exp. Hypertension, Theory Pract.*, A7(9), 1301, 1985. With permission.)

state within 60 sec. At 60 sec of incubation, the SR fractions from the HP-diet and MET-diet animals exhibited Ca^{2+}-binding activities that were significantly higher ($p < 0.001$) than those from the LP and STD diet groups. Oxalate facilitated Ca^{2+} uptake by the SR from various diet groups reached a maximum after 15 sec of incubation time (Figure 3). The Ca^{2+} uptake activity of the SR from the MET-diet group was significantly higher ($p < 0.001$) only than those determined for the other diet groups. Although the Ca^{2+} concentrations required for half-maximal uptake activities ($K_{0.5}$) (Figure 4) were not different amongst the SR from all diet groups, the maximal uptake (B_{max}) activities of the SR from the HP-diet and MET-diet groups of animals were significantly higher ($p < 0.001$) than those of the LP and control (STD) diet groups. This finding would suggest that through mechanism not yet understood, the high protein diets could have unmasked or induced increases in Ca^{2+} binding sites on the SR membranes.

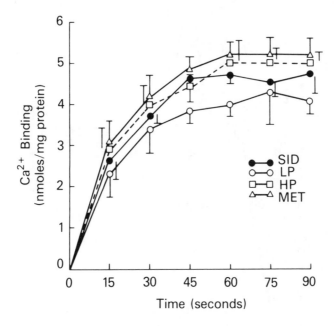

FIGURE 2.   Time course of ⁴⁵Ca²⁺ binding to SR from SHRSP. ⁴⁵Ca²⁺ binding was determined as described in Materials and Methods.[20] Experimental data was compared by analysis of variance followed by student's *t*-test. Each data point represents the mean ± sem of five experiments using separate membrane preparations. At 60 sec, $p < 0.01$ for LP vs. STD, $p < 0.001$ for LP vs. HP, and $p < 0.001$ for LP vs. MET. No significant differences at any other time point and between the other groups. LP = low protein diet, STD = standard diet, HP = high protein diet, and MET = high methionine diet. (Diolulu, M. A., et al., *Clin. Exp. Hypertension, Theory Pract.*, A7(9), 1301, 1985. With permission of Marcel Dekker, Inc.)

DISCUSSION

Certain diets provide protection from the neurological and pathological sequelae that develop in stroke-prone rats.[26] Diets supplemented with either high fish or soybean protein up to 50% of control are effective in preventing stroke in the SHRSP.[29]

The percentages of crude protein and total essential amino acids are 1.3 and 1.4 times, respectively, greater in the American (NIH) diet than in the Japanese diet. Of interest is the higher (1.7 times) content of the essential amino acid methionine in the NIH diet than in the Japanese diet. The inclusion of 1.5% methionine[30] or taurine[18] (a putative metabolite of methionine normally present in large amount in mammalian organs) in drinking water also has been shown to significantly reduce the incidence of stroke in the SHRSP.

The protective mechanism of increased dietary protein and/or methionine on the incidence of stroke is not completely understood at the present time. However, hypertension is a known predisposing factor in stroke in experimental animals. In Wistar-Kyoto rats the BP is in the range of 120 to 150 mmHg and cerebral lesions are seldom evident. The stroke-resistant SHR with BP generally below 200 mmHg exhibits an incidence of stroke of less than 10%. The stroke-prone rats have a BP between 220 and 250 mmHg and exhibit higher (80%) stroke incidence than the SHR.[2,31] In contrast to

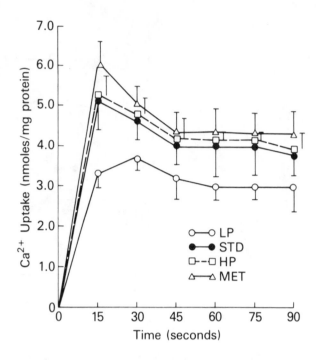

FIGURE 3.   Time course of ATP-dependent, oxalate-facilitated Ca^{2+} Uptake by myocardial SR from SHRSP. $^{45}Ca^{2+}$ uptake was determined as described in Materials and Methods. Experimental data was compared by analysis of variance followed by student's *t*-test. Each data point represents the mean ± sem of five experiments using separate membrane preparations. At 15 sec, $p < 0.001$ for LP vs. MET, $p < 0.001$ for LP vs. HP and $p < 0.005$ for LP vs. STD. At 30 sec, $p < 0.05$ for LP vs. STD, and $p < 0.01$ for LP vs. MET. No other significant differences at any other time point studied. LP = low protein diet, STD = standard diet, HP = high protein diet, and MET = high methionine diet. (Diolulu, M. A., et al., *Clin. Exp. Hypertension, Theory Pract.*, A7(9), 1301, 1985. With permission.)

soybean protein, dietary protein especially of fish source (contains high amount of essential sulfoamino acids) is effective in reducing BP and stroke incidence.[16] It was proposed that a direct effect of sulfoamino acids accounted for the lower BP in animals fed a high protein diet.

The effect of diet on BP also may be due to effects on Ca^{2+} metabolism. The results of the current investigation indicate that in contrast to LP diets, HP and MET diets increase (1) the B_{max} (maximal binding activity) values but not the Ca^{2+} concentration required for half-maximal Ca^{2+} uptake ($K_{0.5}$) and (2) the activity of $(Ca^{2+}\text{-}Mg^{2+})\text{-}AT$-Pase of the SR from SHRSP. It is generally believed that the ATP-dependent Ca^{2+}-binding and accumulating activities of the SR serve as the in vitro manifestation of the Ca^{2+}-pump function of this membrane in vivo. The activity of this membrane pump maintains the cytoplasmic Ca^{2+} concentration in muscle cells at physiological level of below $\sim 10^{-7} M$ thus promoting muscle relaxation.[12] Subcellular membranes of spontaneously hypertensive rats and other models of experimental hypertension exhibit reduced ATP-dependent Ca^{2+} transport activities. This membrane defect may be associated with physiological events leading to hypertension.[8] The biochemical mechanism

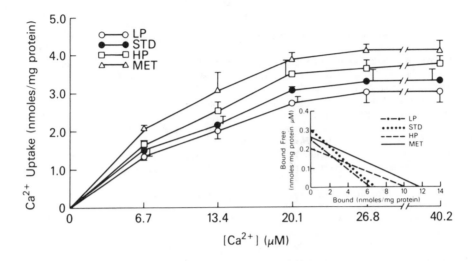

FIGURE 4.   ATP-dependent, oxalate-facilitated $^{45}Ca^{2+}$ uptake by SR from SHRSP at varying Ca^{2+} concentrations. $^{45}Ca^{2+}$ accumulation was determined for 60 sec as described in Materials and Methods. Each data point represents the mean ± sem of five experiments. Inset is Scatchard plot of uptake data. Values for B_{max} and $K_{0.5}$ are presented in Results. LP = low protein diet, STD = standard diet, HP = high protein diet, and MET = high methionine diet. (Diolulu, M. A., et al., *Clin. Exp. Hypertension, Theory Pract.*, A7(9), 1301, 1985. With permission.)

by which HP or methionine supplemented diets reduce BP is not known at the present time. However it is well documented in the literature that the methionine from dietary protein may be utilized for the synthesis of either proteins or S-adenosylmethionine (AdoMet). AdoMet serves as a methyl donor in numerous biological transmethylation reactions such as the conversion of phosphatidylethanolamine (PE) to phosphatidyl-choline (PC).[32,33] The $(Ca^{2+}-Mg^{2+})$-ATPase, which is a key element in the regulatory activity of the SR, constitutes 60 to 80% of the total protein content of the SR. This enzyme is an intrinsic membrane protein that penetrates into the lipid phase of the SR membrane and requires membrane phospholipid for activity.[34] PC-containing lipids support ATPase better than PE lipids whereas maximal Ca^{2+} translocation activity requires both the PC and PE lipids.[35] In addition, results from investigations indicate that in order to be active, membrane proteins need an appropriate lipid environment and that the level of activity increases with the fluidity of the surrounding lipid.[36,37] The fluidity of the cell membrane lipids has been implicated in a number of membrane functions such as enzyme activity[38] and transport.[39] Hoffman et al.[40] proposed that the concentration of AdoMet in the perfused liver is dependent on the availability of me-thionine. Thus, the supply of this amino acid could be of primary importance in the regulation of the conversion of PE to PC. The diet-associated differences in Ca^{2+}-ATPase and Ca^{2+} uptake activities observed in these experiments could reflect possible variations in the lipid environment of the enzyme in the SR from SHRSP. Diet-related improvement in Ca^{2+}-pump activity of the SR from the SHRSP could keep the concen-tration of calcium in the sarcoplasm at a low level. Such an effect would reduce vas-cular contraction and lower peripheral resistance. However, the influence of diet on the physicochemical state of the SR membrane in spontaneously hypertensive rat re-quires further investigation.

REFERENCES

1. Okamoto, K. and Aoki, K., Development of a strain in spontaneously hypertensive rats, *Jpn. Circ. J.*, 27, 282, 1965.
2. Folkow, B., Hallback, M., Lundgren, Y., Sivertsson, R., and Weiss, L., Importance of adaptive changes in vascular design for establishment of primary hypertension, studied in man and in spontaneously hypertensive rats, *Circ. Res.*, 32, 33(Suppl. 1), 2, 1973.
3. Okamoto, K., Nosaka, S., Yamori, Y., and Matsumoto, M., Participation of neural factors in the pathogenesis of hypertension in the spontaneously hypertensive rat, *Jpn. Heart J.*, 8, 168, 1967.
4. Yamori, Y., Contribution of cardiovascular factors to the development of hypertension in spontaneously hypertensive rats, *Jpn. Heart J.*, 15, 194, 1974.
5. Nagatsu, T., Kato, T., Numata, Y., Ikuta, K., Umeazwa, H., Matsuzaki, M., and Takeuchi, T., Serum dopamine-β-hydroxylase activity in developing hypertensive rats, *Nature (London)*, 251, 630, 1974.
6. Ichijima, K., Morphological studies on the peripheral small arteries of spontaneously hypertensive rats, *Jpn. Circ. J.*, 33, 785, 1969.
7. Folkow, B., Hallback, M., Lundgren, Y., and Weiss, L., Background of increased flow resistance and vascular reactivity in spontaneously hypertensive rats, *Acta Physiol. Scand.*, 80, 93, 1970.
8. Kwan, C.-Y. and Daniel, E. E., Calcium transport by plasma membrane vesicles isolated from vascular smooth muscle of normal and hypertensive rats, in *Vasodilation*, Vanhoutte, P. M. and Lensen, I., Eds., Raven Press, New York, 1981, 405.
9. Bohr, D. F. and Sitrin, M., Regulation of vascular smooth muscle contraction: changes in experimental hypertension, *Circ. Res.*, 27 (Suppl. 2), 83, 1970.
10. Wei, F., Janis, R. A., and Daniel, E. E., Studies on subcellular fractions from mesenteric arteries of spontaneously hypertensive rats: alterations of both calcium uptake and enzyme activities, *Blood Vessels*, 13, 293, 1976.
11. Ito, Y. and Chidsey, C. A., Intracellular calcium and myocardial contractility. IV. Distribution of calcium in the failing canine heart, *J. Mol. Cell. Cardiol.*, 4, 507, 1972.
12. Tada, M., Yamamoto, T., and Tonomura, Y., Molecular mechanism of active calcium transport by sarcoplasmic reticulum, *Physiol. Rev.*, 58, 1, 1978.
13. Yamori, Y., Neurogenic mechanisms of spontaneous hypertension, in *Regulation of Blood Pressure by the Central Nervous System*, Onesti, G., Fernandes, M., and Kim, K. E., Eds., Grune and Stratton, New York, 1976, 65.
14. Yamori, Y., Neural and nonneural mechanisms in spontaneous hypertension, *Clin. Sci. Mol. Med.*, 51, 431s, 1976.
15. Yamori, Y., Pathogenesis of spontaneous hypertension as a model for essential hypertension, *Jpn. Circ. J.*, 41, 259, 1977.
16. Yamori, Y., Horie, R., Ikeda, K., Nara, Y., and Lovenberg, W., Prophylactic effect of dietary protein on stroke and its mechanisms, in *Prophylactic Approach to Hypertensive Diseases*, Yamori, Y., Lovenberg, W., and Fries, E. O., Eds., Raven Press, New York, 1979, 497.
17. Yamori, Y., Horie, R., Akiguchi, I., Nara, Y., Ohtaka, M., and Fukase, M., Pathogenetic mechanism of stroke in stroke-prone SHR, in *Progress in Brain Research, Vol. 47: Hypertension and Brain Mechanisms*, de Jong, W., Ed., Elsevier, Amsterdam, 219, 1977.
18. Nara, Y., Yamori, Y., and Lovenberg, W., Effect of dietary taurine on blood pressure in genetically hypertensive rats, *Biochem. Pharmacol.*, 27, 2689, 1978.
19. Page, I. H., The long slow road to progress: A lesson in humility, in *Fundamental fault in hypertension*, Sambhi, M. P., Ed., Martius Nijhoff, 1984. 3.
20. Hasselbach, W., Relaxing factor and the relaxation of muscle, *Prog. Biophys. Mol. Biol.*, 14, 167, 1965.
21. Bohr, D. F., Vascular smooth muscle: Dual effect of calcium, *Science*, 139, 597, 1963.
22. Postnov, Y. V., Orlov, S. N., and Pokndin, N. I., Decrease of calcium binding by the red blood cell membrane in spontaneously hypertensive rats and in essential hypertension, *Pflugers Arch.*, 379, 191, 1979.
23. WHO Expert Committee on Arterial Hypertension, Arterial hypertension. Technical Report Series 628, World Health Organization, Rome, 1978.
24. Knapka, J. J., Smith, K. P., and Judge, F. J., Effect of open and closed formula rations on the performance of three strains of laboratory mice, *Lab. Anim. Sci.*, 24, 480, 1974.
25. Diolulu, M. A., Buck, S. H., Knapka, J., and Lovenberg, W., ATP-dependent calcium uptake in myocardial sarcoplasmic reticulum from spontaneously hypertensive rats: effect of modification of dietary protein, *Clin. Exp. Hypertension*, A7(9), 1301, 1985.

26. Yamori, Y., Horie, R., Tanase, H., Fujiwara, K., Nara, Y., and Lovenberg, W., Possible role of nutritional factors in the incidence of cerebral lesions in stroke-prone spontaneously hypertensive rats, *Hypertension,* 6, 49, 1984.

27. Harigaya, S. and Schwartz, A., Rate of calcium binding and uptake in normal animal and failing human cardiac muscle: membrane vesicles (relaxing system) and mitrochondria, *Circ. Res.,* 25, 781, 1969.

28. MacLennau, D. H. and Holland, P. C., The calcium transport ATPase of sarcoplasmic reticulum, in *The Enzymes of Biological Membranes: Membrane Transport,* Martonosi, A., Ed., Plenum Press, New York, 1976, 221.

29. Yamori, Y., Horie, R., Handa, H., Ohtaka, M., Nara, Y., Fukaske, M., Pathogenetic approach to the prophylaxis of stroke and atherogenesis in SHR spontaneous hypertension, in *DHEW Publication No. (NIH) 77-1179,* Washington, D.C., Department of Health, Education, and Welfare, 1977, 269.

30. Yamori, Y., Horie, R., Nara, Y., Kihara, M., and Ikeda, K., Abstracts, *Eighth Int. Cong. Pharmacol.,* Tokyo, 1981, 234.

31. Okamoto, K., Yamori, Y., and Nagaoka, H., Establishment of the stroke-prone spontaneously hypertensive rats, *Circ. Res.,* (Suppl. 1), 143, 1974.

32. Hirata, F., Axelrod, J., and Strittmatter, W. J., Methylation of membrane phospholipids, in *Transmethylation,* Vol. 5, Usdin, E., Borchardt, R. T., and Creveling, C. R., Eds., Elsevier, Amsterdam, 1979, 233.

33. Finkelstein, J. D., Regulation of methionine metabolism in mammals, in *Transmethylation,* Vol. 5, Usdin, E., Borchardt, R. T., and Creveling, C. R., Eds., Elsevier, Amsterdam, 1979, 49.

34. Martonisi, A., Donley, J., and Halpin, R. A., Sarcoplasmic reticulum. III. The role of phospholipids in the adenosine triphosphatase activity and Ca^{2+} transport, *J. Biol. Chem.,* 243, 61, 1968.

35. Knowles, A. F., Eytan, E., and Racker, E., Phospholipid-protein interactions in the Ca^{2+}-adenosine triphosphatase of sarcoplasmic reticulum, *J. Biol. Chem.,* 251, 5161, 1976.

36. Sanderman, H., Regulation of membrane enzymes by lipids, *Biochim. Biophys. Acta,* 515, 209, 1978.

37. Silvius, J. R. and McElhaney, R. N., Membrane lipid physical state and modulation of the Na^+-Mg^{2+}-ATPase activity in *Acholeplasma laidlawii* B, *Proc. Natl. Acad. Sci. U.S.A.,* 77, 1255, 1980.

38. Kimelberg, H. K., Alterations in phospholipid-dependent ($Na^+ + K^+$)-ATPase activity due to lipid fluidity. Effects of cholesterol and Mg^{2+}, *Biochim. Biophys. Acta,* 413, 143, 1975.

39. Overath, P., Schairer, H. U., and Stoffel, W., Correlation of in vivo and in vitro phase transitions of membrane lipids in *Escherichia coli, Proc. Natl. Acad. Sci. U.S.A.,* 67, 606, 1970.

40. Hoffman, D. R., Marion, D. W., Cornatzer, W. E., and Duerre, J. A., S-adenosylmethionine and S-adenosylhomocysteine metabolism is isolated rat liver: effects of L-methionine, L-homocysteine and adenosine, *J. Biol. Chem.,* 255, 10822, 1980.

Chapter 9

NUTRITIONAL AND PATHOLOGICAL ASPECTS OF ATHEROSCLEROSIS IN AGING ADULTS

Miguel A. Guzman and Jack P. Strong

TABLE OF CONTENTS

I. GENERAL BACKGROUND

At the turn of the century, infectious diseases were the major contributors to human mortality. At that time coronary heart disease (CHD) and myocardial infarction, its principal clinical manifestation, were rare medical entities that were not commonly reported.[1] With the gradual and successful control of infections and the first objective description of myocardial infarction in 1912,[2] the situation changed and CHD was recognized and reported with ever increasing frequency, especially among the more affluent white men in Europe and the U.S.[3,4]

By the time of World War II, CHD was the leading cause of death in various countries and geographic locations.[2] In the U.S., the frequency of CHD continued to increase through the decade of the 1950s, achieving epidemic proportions by the end of the decade and early 1960s.[2,3] The same trend was apparent in many, but not all, industrialized nations. This is well illustrated by data available for Japan for the same period of time[5,6] documenting, for this industrialized nation, a CHD morbidity and mortality more in line with the generally lower rates commonly reported in nonindustrialized developing nations.[7] By the mid 1960s, CHD mortality apparently had reached its peak in the U.S., but even after a definite declining trend was well established by 1970,[8,9] CHD continued to be the leading cause of death in this country.[10,11] Also, and as could be expected, the decreasing trend in mortality was not uniform within the country but occurred preferentially by regions.[2,4,12] A decline in CHD mortality, similar to the one observed in the U.S. from 1969 to 1977, has been reported presently in several other industrialized nations.[2]

There is abundant evidence of a high correlation between the severity and extent of coronary atherosclerosis and CHD[13,14] suggesting, as is commonly believed, that coronary atherosclerosis provides the basis for the development of CHD.[2,4,15] Autopsy studies show that the extent and severity of atherosclerosis not only differ among individuals and populations[16] but may also differ through time within a given population as a result of changes in the environment and lifestyles.[17] The physiopathologic process that leads to atherosclerosis is not completely understood but it is generally agreed that the process begins very early in life[15,18,19] and develops slowly through time without readily apparent clinical manifestations[2] until narrowing or occlusion of the coronary arteries produces ischemia to the myocardium. In the early stages, often before age 15, atherogenesis affects the intima of the coronary arteries with deposition of fat, mainly cholesterol ester, and increased cellularity. Connective tissue proliferation, in reaction to the fat deposits, leads to the formation of thickened plaques (fibrous plaques). After a period of time, usually measured in decades, as a result of atherosclerotic plaques growing and obstructing normal coronary blood flow through reduction of the arterial lumen, and with the added complications of rupture of the plaque and thrombus formation, the common symptoms of coronary atherosclerosis (sudden death, myocardial infarction, angina) appear suddenly.[11,20-22] The critical aspect in this process is the fact that the first sign of existing underlying CHD is death, often occurring before any therapy can be initiated.[21,22] Accordingly, efforts for conquering CHD, without neglecting treatment, must be directed preferentially to prevention. In this effort, the identification of appropriate target factors — factors associated with the underlying atherosclerotic process and high risk of CHD — is essential.

II. RISK FACTORS, CHD, AND ATHEROSCLEROSIS

In a strict sense, a "risk factor" for CHD should be shown to be associated with the disease and also demonstrated to assist in predicting the probability of appearance of

CHD based on measured levels of the factor. A causal relation is not required and an association established through prospective studies suffices to identify a "risk factor". The term "risk factor", however, has been popularized and is used to include practically any associate of CHD. Under these conditions, whenever a disease differs in frequency through time, between cultures or geographic locations, there is opportunity for investigation of possible causes of the disease and the identification of associate factors that may contribute to the risk of contracting the disease.[3,4]

The population differences in CHD frequency (morbidity and mortality) described in the preceding paragraphs have stimulated abundant research of the disease. These studies have made it clear that CHD is not a random occurrence and cases differ from comparable normal controls in a number of personal traits and habits related to lifestyle which are, therefore, believed associated with increased risk of CHD.[11,23,24] Thus, age, male sex, elevated serum lipids (particularly cholesterol), hypertension, cigarette smoking, hyperglycemia (diabetes), obesity, sedentary living (lack of exercise), psychosocial tension, and history of premature atherosclerosis, among others, are most commonly associated with increased risk of CHD.[24,25]

As a result of epidemiological studies[22,26,27] and observations made during normal times and during periods of circumstantial food restrictions,[28,29] at present there is agreement that diet is associated with CHD. It remains uncertain, however, how diet, as risk factor, may relate to the development of atherosclerosis and CHD.[30] Nevertheless, if atherosclerotic lesions are important in establishing CHD risk, as is commonly believed,[15] the investigation of diet-lesion relations will contribute valuable information for elucidating the potential role of food and nutrients in the etiology of CHD with identification of nutrition related risk factors.

III. DIET AND ATHEROSCLEROTIC LESIONS

Methods for evaluating atherosclerosis in the living population provide information only on very advanced lesions which significantly have narrowed the arterial lumen.[24] This may limit the range of lesion quantitation sufficiently as to preclude proper evaluation of risk factors. Lacking the technology required for sensitive full range quantitation of the extent of atherosclerotic lesions in living subjects, information on risk factor-lesion associations has been obtained through autopsy studies.[24,30] Autopsy studies have inherent well-recognized limitations[31] and in the case of risk factor investigations, the selection bias of autopsied cases may also either obscure true relations or produce spurious associations.[32,33] At present, however, autopsies provide the only way to measure lesions within the arterial wall[34,35] with the accuracy required for studies of their association with suspected risk factors. This review will focus attention on a sample of such autopsy studies, presenting an overview of their findings.

A. The International Atherosclerosis Project
Epidemiologic studies have consistently demonstrated significant correlations between the intakes of cholesterol, total fat, saturated fat, calories, and CHD mortalitations of atherosclerotic lesions using a standardized reliable visual method[37,38] on centrally prepared arterial specimens (aorta and coronary arteries), collected at the time of atuopsy by uniform procedures[39] in 15 laboratories, representing 14 countries and 19 distinct location-race groups.

This extensive international evaluation of atherosclerotic lesions afforded, for the first time, a unique opportunity to test in a human autopsy sample, current hypotheses of the relationships of dietary variables with atherosclerotic lesions. The association of an index of lesion involvement, generated from the IAP results,[16] with nutrition related variables, as reported in diet surveys of the living populations from which the autopsied cases in the IAP were drawn, was examined using rank correlation methods.[40] The results showed significant positive correlations of the lesion index with serum cholesterol levels (r = 0.755) and with percent calories from fat (r = 0.668). The rank correlations of the lesion index with two other nutrition related variables, percent animal fat in total fat and total amount of sugar consumed, were small and without significance. A strong positive correlation of animal protein consumption with the lesion index was also observed but it was not considered etiologically important since this dietary variable, in the populations considered, closely paralleled fat calories and also because of the dominant role generally attributed to fat intake in determining levels of serum cholesterol, severity of atherosclerosis, and incidence of CHD.[40]

B. The New Orleans Autopsy Studies

A case-related analytical approach, based on measures of lesions and diet in the same individual, may be more appropriate for detecting associations of diet related factors with atherosclerosis. The New Orleans sample collected late in the IAP and a sample of arterial specimens collected subsequently for studies of the relationship of cigarette smoking with atherosclerosis,[41,42] provided a unique opportunity to extend, on a case-related basis, the earlier incipient IAP exploration of diet-atherosclerosis associations. These studies now will be described in some detail.

1. Methodology

The collection and processing of specimens and the evaluation of atherosclerotic lesions followed the extensively tested methods used in the IAP.[37,38] The measure of atherosclerosis chosen for these case-related dietary studies was the average of the percent of intimal surface of the three main coronary arteries involved with raised lesions (fibrous plaques, complicated and calcified lesions combined).[37] For the corresponding required assessments of dietary lifestyles (eating pattern and nutrient intake), however, it was necessary to develop, test, and validate appropriate methodology for the collection of information to be provided posthumously by a surviving close associate of the deceased. Methodological investigations demonstrated that it is possible to obtain reliable qualitative and quantitative estimates of the usual 28-day pattern of food intake during the terminal year of life of a deceased adult man through information obtained by questioning a consenting surviving female associate.[43] To qualify as informant, however, this associate had to satisfy three conditions: (1) the associate must have shared the same household with the deceased man for at least 1 year prior to his death; (2) the associate bought, prepared, and served the food eaten by the subject; and (3) for detailed nutrient studies, the deceased, while alive, must have eaten two thirds of his meals in the home. In the course of testing this methodology, it was noted also that the use of locally valid food models in the course of diet questioning interviews, reduced the range of variability of the estimates of food intake over all foods, to approximately one half of that observed under similar conditions without the assistance of the food models.[44] An updated extended table of nutrient values[45] was used for the conversion of the quantitated food intakes into estimates of daily intake of nutrients.

Within the frame of reference established by the conditions outlined, the investigators were able to identify 456 surviving associates of autopsied men aged 20 to 60 years, who qualified as informants for the investigation of the eating pattern of the deceased men during the year preceeding their death; 253 of these deceased men also had eaten two thirds of their meals at home, thus satisfying the established conditions for inclusion in detailed studies for the estimation of their daily nutrient intake from information rendered by their respective qualified and consenting surviving associates.[46,47]

2. Eating Pattern, Related Variables, and Atherosclerosis

The eating pattern of the 456 autopsied men, while alive, was fairly stable since 71% of their associate informants indicated that only minor diet changes had occurred through time. In a typical day, these men slept 8 hr, ate 3 meals and 3 snacks, smoked 20 cigarettes, drank one alcoholic beverage, and consumed 3 to 4 caffeine-containing drinks,[46] reflecting a similar general lifestyle pattern to that previously described in living populations from New Orleans using the same methodology.[43] The general pattern of coronary raised lesions by age and race in this autopsy sample also was similar to that previously reported for New Orleans in the IAP.[16]

Preliminary investigation of lesion associations showed age, race, and occupation as the strongest primary correlates of coronary raised lesions involvement. Cigarette smoking rate during the 10 years preceding death and the frequency of caffeine-containing beverages, also were identified as significant primary correlates of lesions, and these two variables, in turn, correlated significantly with seven other highly intercorrelated eating pattern variables.[46]

A stepwise discriminant function analysis approach was used next in these investigations[46] to try to identify, from a set of selected eating pattern variables, those which may best assist in distinguishing between high and low atherosclerotic involvement populations. The reference populations for these analyses were the upper and lower quartiles in the age-adjusted distribution of coronary lesion involvement. The stepwise construction of various discriminant functions for the 239 cases with complete information for inclusion in these analyses, in general, selected eating pattern and related variables for a significant improvement of the discriminating power of these functions in the following order: number of meals and heavy snacks, frequency of caffeine drinks (with or without sugar), frequency of alcohol, cigarette smoking rate during the 10 years preceding death, and ingestion span. The sequence in variable selection, as an indicator of relative importance in aiding in the discrimination between high and low raised coronary lesion populations, was the item of interest in the discriminant function analyses. The results described were interpreted by the investigators as an indication that not only what is eaten but also the manner of eating, may play a role in the development and progression of atherosclerosis and its complications.[46]

In parallel with these case-related findings, pertaining to the association of eating pattern variables with coronary atherosclerosis in an autopsy sample, other investigators have reported associations of eating pattern variables with myocardial infarction,[48] death due to CHD,[49] and risk of CHD.[50] Frequency of eating, nibbling, and gorging also have been reported as associates of lipogenesis[51] and adiposity in adult men and women[52] which, in turn, are associates of obesity, a condition often reported as a CHD risk factor.[25,53,54]

3. Nutrient Intake and Atherosclerosis

For these studies, 28-day eating pattern food frequency data, quantitated with the aid of food models, were converted into individual estimates of daily nutrient intakes of each of 253 deceased men, 20 to 60 years of age, with surviving female associates who qualified as respondents for detailed diet studies.[43,47] On the average, these respondents had shared the household with the now-deceased subject for a period of 18 years prior to the occurrence of the death.[47]

The nutrient intake estimates for each subject were merged with the independently determined visual estimate of the percent of intimal surface of the three main branches of the coronary arteries involved with raised lesions,[37] the measure of atherosclerosis selected for use in the case-related exploration of associations with diet variables. The 253 diet-atherosclerosis records, complete with demographic data, were distributed

Table 1
MEAN PERCENT OF CORONARY INTIMA
WITH RAISED LESIONS (RL) IN TERTILE
GROUPS DEFINED BY CALORIE-RELATED
INTAKES OF VARIOUS NUTRIENTS — THE
NEW ORLEANS AUTOPSY STUDIES[46,55]

Nutrient	Tertile groupings by nutrient intake		
	Lower (84) % RL	Middle (85) % RL	Upper (84) % RL
Animal protein	26	29	39
Vegetable protein	39	30	25
Lysine	29	27	38
Total fat	25	35	35
Myristic acid	27	28	39
Oleic acid	25	35	34
Starch	42	29	23
Fructose	24	31	39
Thiamine	41	26	27
Riboflavin	26	30	38
Niacin	24	28	43
Calcium	25	33	37
Sodium	40	30	25
Iodine	24	32	28

Note: Figures in parentheses specify the number of cases.

into tertile groups based on the distribution of daily intakes for each nutrient, thus generating as many sets of tertile groupings as there were nutrients in the data records. Each set included 84, 85, and 84 subjects in the lower, middle, and upper tertile groups, respectively.

The analytical basis in these studies was the comparison of the raised lesion involvement among tertile groups for a given nutrient, using analysis of variance techniques to detect increasing or decreasing trends, after establishing that the composition of each nutrient tertile grouping under consideration was not age or race dependent, since these two characteristics consistently have been shown to be related to lesions.[16] All estimates of intake were expressed on a calorie-related basis to reduce distortions that may result from large individual differences in calorie intake.[47] The results of the comparison of the percent coronary raised lesions among the intake tertile groupings for the 47 dietary components considered in these analyses, identified 14 nutrients associated with apparent significant trends in lesions.[47,55] A summary of these findings is presented in Table 1.

The observed positive association of animal protein intake with lesions, considered in conjunction with the negative association of intake of vegetable protein and starch with lesions, is interpreted by the investigators as an indication that a greater consumption of foods of vegetal origin may be beneficial in providing protection against atherosclerosis.[47,55] Although short of significance, the observed tendency toward lesser lesions with increasing fiber content in the usual diet of the men included in these studies also supports this hypothesis. In this connection, the results described in these case-related diet-lesion studies on deceased men agree with results from studies of living subjects which have associated a higher consumption of foods of plant origin, particularly starch, with lower serum cholesterol levels,[56,57] a desirable condition generally recognized as conducive to lesser atherosclerosis, and CHD.[11,22,24-27] Whether this beneficial effect is a consequence of specific elements that are characteristic of plant foods, or simply the result of corresponding compensating lesser intakes of rich foods of animal origin, is a question that merits investigation. Presently, however, studies using animal models suggest that proteins of vegetal and animal origin, per se, contribute differently in atherogenesis.[58,59]

Some of the more specific nutrient-lesion associations identified in this study may be the result of primary dietary internutrient associations. Thus, the positive association of lysine, riboflavin, calcium, and iodine with lesions may well be a consequence of the fact that, in general, foods of animal origin are the main source of these nutrients. Similarly, the negative association of sodium with lesions may reflect an effect of carriers — legumes, vegetables, and starchy foods — since generous amounts of salt are commonly used in the New Orleans area in cooking foods of plant origin.[55] The apparent association of niacin intake with lesions may be an indirect result of the positive association of raised coronary lesions with the frequency of intake of caffeine-containing drinks, mainly coffee,[46,48] given the reported high content of niacin in coffee.[55,60]

The positive association of the intake of myristic acid with lesions is consistent with findings that identify a high intake of saturated fats as an index of high risk of CHD[11,22,25,26] because of the association of these fats, and particularly of myristic acid,[61] with elevated serum cholesterol. In this connection, Moore, et al.[55] also mention a positive but not significant association of the intakes of two other saturated fatty acids (palmitic and stearic) with raised coronary lesions. The positive association of the intake of the monounsaturated oleic acid with lesions, was attributed to a reflection of the overall positive association of the total fat intake with lesions previously reported by these investigators.[47,55] Finally, the apparent relation of the intake of fructose (positive) and of thiamine (negative) with lesions cannot be explained in terms of known nutrient and food source associations.[55]

An effort to relate these nutrient findings to the original food sources[62] to explore possible associations of market foods with lesions had only limited success; the results, however, supported the general conclusion that an increased consumption of foods of vegetal origin, often associated with lower intakes of fat, particularly saturated fat, may relate to a decreased atherosclerotic involvement in the coronary arteries.[46,53,55] This finding supports a similar general conclusion proposed by other investigators as a result of observations derived from epidemiological studies in living populations.[22,27]

C. The Puerto Rico Heart Health Program

The Puerto Rico Heart Health Program (PRHHP) is a long-term prospective epidemiological survey, initiated in 1965 for the purpose of studying the association of potential risk factors with the prevalence and incidence of CHD. It was designed to cover a target population of 10,000 men, 45 to 64 years of age, residents of three urban and four rural municipalities located in a geographic radius of 25 miles in the vicinity of San Juan.[63] Social, dietary, and medical histories as well as physical examinations, electrocardiograms, and blood lipid determinations were obtained for each subject admitted to the study, using standardized procedures and appropriate measures of quality control. Of 9824 men initially examined, 8793 were in the desired age range and 8254 of them were considered to be free of CHD at the time of the basal examination.[63] Reexamination cycles in the PRHHP were scheduled at intervals of 2½ to 3 years.[64]

1. Methodology

The method of 24-hr recall was used to obtain the diet history information for each subject during the first examination cycle implemented from 1965 to 1968. Trained dieticians recorded and coded the food intake information of each subject interviewed.

This information was converted into estimates of daily nutrient intakes using a specially constructed food composition table, based on standard references considered appropriate for Puerto Rico.[65]

There were 970 deaths recorded among participants in the PRHHP between 1965 and 1977. The routine autopsy rate for Puerto Rico during this period was approximately 40%, however, and mainly because of difficulties in identifying decedents as members of the study cohort, only 139 autopsies were evaluated under the special procedures and conditions established by the study protocol.[35]

The collection and processing of arterial specimens and the evaluation of atherosclerotic lesions followed the IAP procedures.[37,38] For each case, the three main branches of the coronary arteries and two segments of the aorta (thoracic and abdominal) were graded for extent of atherosclerosis by the experienced grading team (five pathologists) of the Department of Pathology of the Louisiana State University Medical Center in New Orleans, La. All gradings were performed without reference to either demographic information or clinical and pathological findings. The percent of intimal surface involved with raised lesions, the measure of atherosclerosis used in the New Orleans studies described in the preceding section of this review, was also selected as the measure of atherosclerosis in the Puerto Rico study of associations of diet with lesions.[35] The prospective nature of the PRHHP however, additionally provided an opportunity for a parallel examination of associations between diet and serum lipids[65] and also between diet and CHD.[57]

2. Diet and Atherosclerosis

The 139 protocol autopsy deaths did not differ in terms of urban-rural composition from the 831 deaths that were not autopsied. The protocol autopsy deaths, however, included a greater proportion of cancer deaths (8 vs 25%) than the group of deaths that was not autopsied. Comparison of 18 characteristics between the two groups of deaths (autopsied and not autopsied) did not suggest a serious selection bias in the process of obtaining the protocol autopsies.[35]

The associations of raised lesions with 18 antemortem factors, which included four dietary intake variables, were investigated by simple correlation analysis. The product moment correlation coefficient of each antemortem factor with the estimate of raised lesions for the combined coronary arteries and also for the combined segments of the aorta, was calculated using the total group of protocol autopsies and also the segregated urban and rural subclasses. Additionally, antemortem factor-raised lesion correlations were calculated in a subgroup of subjects from the urban and rural locations of the study who died of noncardiovascular causes.

The simple correlation coefficients of coronary and aortic raised lesions with systolic blood pressure (BP), serum cholesterol, and the intakes of calories, total fat, starch, and alcohol (the only four dietary variables considered by these investigators) are presented for various case groupings in Table 2. These results clearly identify serum cholesterol as the strongest and most consistent positive correlate of lesions in both the coronary arteries and aorta for all the case groupings considered. Systolic BP also appears as a strong correlate of raised lesions, particularly in the group of noncardiovascular deaths. The calculated correlations of raised lesions with the diet variables are generally smaller than those described for the association of lesions with serum cholesterol and systolic BP. These correlations, however, are uniformly negative in both the coronary arteries and aorta in all case groupings considered. While the negative associations of the intakes of calories, starch and alcohol agree with results of other investigators,[46,47] the apparent negative relation of total fat intake with lesions is puzzling and contrary to expectations. The total fat intake of the men in this autopsy sample,

Table 2
SIMPLE CORRELATION COEFFICIENTS OF CORONARY AND
AORTIC RAISED LESIONS WITH SELECTED ANTEMORTEM
CHARACTERISTICS — THE PUERTO RICO HEART HEALTH
PROGRAM[35]

Antemortem characteristic	Coronary arteries				Aorta			
	Total (139)	Rural (36)	Urban (103)	NCVD (54)	Total (120)	Rural (31)	Urban (89)	NCVD (45)
Systolic pressure	.22	.07	.30	.38	.25	.27	.24	.49
Serum cholesterol	.42	.59	.38	.35	.29	.36	.28	.34
Calorie intake	−.14	−.43	−.07	−.19	−.24	−.55	−.12	−.27
Total fat intake	−.04	−.29	.03	−.13	−.19	−.49	−.11	−.21
Starch intake	−.17	−.29	−.09	−.25	−.19	−.45	−.07	−.26
Alcohol intake	−.10	−.10	−.13	.01	−.18	−.39	−.18	−.24

Note: NCVD = Noncardiovascular deaths. Figures in parentheses specify the number of cases.

particularly among the rural dwellers, however, is lower than that reported for similar populations in the U.S., especially with reference to saturated fatty acids.[65] Conditions resulting from nutritional deficiencies and malabsorption in the population studied, may help in explaining the negative association of total fat intake with lesions reported by these investigators. This observation merits further investigation.

Results of multiple regression analyses did not contribute additional information and relationships in this multivariate setting are similar to those identified bivariately.[35] In summing up the interpretation of their results, the investigators stated: "the results from this study, along with those from other clinical pathologic investigations, lend support to the conclusion that the major cardiovascular risk factors operate through an increase in the atherosclerotic process."[35]

3. Diet, Serum Lipids, and CHD

The 24-hr recall baseline estimates of the nutrient intake of the 8254 participants in the PRHHP, judged to be free of CHD upon admission to the study, were used to investigate possible associations of dietary variables with serum cholesterol and fasting triglycerides.[65] The estimates of nutrient intake were employed also to explore relationships between dietary intake and subsequent incidence of CHD.[57] The nutrients and diet related variables considered in these analyses included: calories, total protein, total fat, saturated fatty acids, monounsaturated fatty acids, polyunsaturated fatty acids, total carbohydrates, starch, refined sugar (sucrose), other carbohydrates, alcohol, cholesterol, caffeine, P:S ratio, and a "salt index".[57,65]

The simple correlation coefficients of the two blood lipid variables (serum cholesterol and triglycerides) with the diet related variables were small, never greater than 0.15, in the two age groups considered (45 to 54 and 55 to 64 years) among the rural and urban residents in the PRHHP. As the investigators point out,[65] such results are practically useless for demonstrating meaningful within group correlations of dietary variables with serum lipid values. Under these conditions a regression analysis approach may be more informative. The correlation analyses, however, identified an apparent association of serum lipids with relative weight, suggesting that this variable should be considered in further explorations of the possible association of blood lipids with diet related variables. Accordingly, the two blood lipids were regressed on each specific diet variable and relative weight, and the diet variable regression coefficient then used to assess the association of each diet variable with the blood lipid under consideration, after compensating for relative weight.

Using the approach described above, Garcia-Palmieri et al.[65] identified the following serum cholesterol associates among the diet related variables included in the study of the urban cohort: percent calories from protein (+), from total fat (+), and from starch (−); dietary cholesterol was a positive associate, while percent carbohydrate from starch was negatively related to serum cholesterol. A similar analysis for the rural cohort did not show the consistency of associations evident in the urban group. The regression analysis for the log transform (to correct skewdness in the distribution) of serum triglycerides on diet related variables and relative weight, revealed only a negative relationship of this blood lipid with the percent of carbohydrate from starch in the urban cohort.

The association of selected dietary variables, measured at the time of baseline examinations, and the incidence of CHD over a 6-year period was examined using a multiple logistic model. The diet variables described above, expressed as absolute age-adjusted mean values[57] were included in these analyses.

The results showed that urban men had significantly higher intakes of total fat and cholesterol than rural men; the urban men also were higher in serum cholesterol values. The rural men, on the other hand, had a higher intake of carbohydrate, particularly starch from rice and beans and the traditional tropical Puerto Rican root vegetables; they also experienced a lower CHD mortality in the 6-year period than the urban men. A significantly lower intake of calories and carbohydrate was associated with the urban men who experienced myocardial infarction or suffered a CHD death; the same association, although not significant, was observed in the rural group of men. Results of a multivariate analysis, which included relative weight, hematocrit, BP, serum cholesterol, alcohol intake, cigarette smoking, place of residence, and age, suggest an inverse association of the intake of carbohydrate from legumes with the incidence of CHD.[57]

Taken together, the results of the PRHHP which identify associations of diet related variables with atherosclerosis, serum lipids, and CHD are generally consistent in suggesting that lower intakes of fat, particularly saturated fats, and higher intakes of complex carbohydrates have a beneficial effect in terms of lower serum cholesterol values, less atherosclerosis, and lower incidence of CHD.

D. The Honolulu Heart Study

The Honolulu Heart Study (HHS) is one of three coordinated cohort studies included in a prospective investigation of cardiovascular disease in native and migrant Japanese men. Because of the geographic locations covered — Japan (Nippon), Honolulu, and San Francisco — the tripartite investigation has been identified in the literature as the NI-HON-SAN study, an acronym which may be freely translated as "the Japanese three".[66] As general background we will describe some results of baseline data comparisons in the NI-HON-SAN study but, for this review, we will focus attention on results from the HHS cohort follow-up studies.

1. Methodology

The procedures for the identification of the men to be included in the cohort studies followed a similar pattern in the three locations — access to an official local roster of individuals to serve as frame of reference for the identification of potential participants, with follow-up to establish personal contact with each candidate for obtaining their consent to participate in the study and initiation of baseline examinations.[66] In Honolulu, 14,426 men born between 1900 and 1919 were identified through Selective Service records from World War II; 11,148 of these men were current residents on

Oahu. When contacted, 9,878 of the residents responded, and during the period 1965 to 1968, individual examinations for baseline data were completed for a total of 8,006 men. The corresponding cohorts in Japan and San Francisco included 2,183 and 2,296 men, respectively.

Each subject completed a questionnaire providing basic demographic and socioeconomic data, a self-assessment of his current health status with descriptions of physical activity, smoking history, and general eating habits. Detailed information on the family and past medical history, with particular attention to cardiovascular events, was obtained at the time of direct examination. At this time, anthropometric measurements, BP, vital capacity, and a standard 12-lead electrocardiogram were determined and recorded. Blood samples were collected for blood group, hematocrit, glucose, uric acid, cholesterol, and triglyceride determinations.[66]

The baseline examination included a dietary interview, conducted by qualified dietitians, to obtain data to evaluate individual diets by the 24-hr recall method. Food models and samples of serving utensils were used as an aid for the quantitation and coding of food intakes as required for their conversion into estimates of nutrient intakes using the food table especially constructed for these studies.[66-69]

Autopsy studies on participants who die during the study period are performed, whenever possible, according to a common protocol. Autopsy studies were not undertaken in California because of the wide dispersion of hospitals serving the Japanese population in this geographic location.[5] In Honolulu, specifically, cohort deaths are ascertained through daily examination of obituary columns and a systematic surveillance of death certificates. Study personnel contact daily the local mortuaries, hospitals, and the office of the Medical Examiner to detect impending autopsies of study subjects and make arrangements to obtain the heart and aorta for standardized dissection and evaluation.[34] At yearly intervals, one of the project investigators evaluates the extent of atherosclerosis on the accumulated collection of arterial specimens using the panel method of the American Heart Association,[70] without reference to other autopsy or clinical findings.[34]

2. Interstudy Baseline Comparisons

The Japanese men in Honolulu are reported to have a higher rate of CHD than their counterparts in Japan, but such rate still remains below that reported for white men in the U.S.[34] Results of the initial examinations for this prospective study also show that the cohort of men living in Japan, a population generally acknowledged to have a low risk of CHD,[6,7,25] differs in many ways from migrant Japanese living in Honolulu and the San Francisco area in California.[66]

The Japanese-American men in Honolulu and San Francisco are approximately 2 cm taller than Japanese men living in Japan. The migrant Japanese also are 8 to 9 kg heavier than the native Japanese. The skinfold measurements on these men conform with the trends in weight, suggesting that the observed weight difference results primarily from differences in adiposity.[66] The migrant Japanese, however, apparently also have a slightly larger body frame as indicated by larger bi-iliac and biacromial diameters. The latter difference is somewhat more apparent at younger ages, while the former does not appear to change with age. A higher vital capacity determined in the California cohort may be a consequence of methodological differences. In Japan and Hawaii ventilation was determined using a Collins Spirometer with manual measurement, while in California, ventilation was measured using a wedge spirometer coupled directly to a computer. The investigators point out that expressing the vital capacity results in relative terms reduces but does not eliminate the observed difference.[66]

BP values in Hawaii and Japan are nearly alike and lower in these two cohorts than in the California cohort. The ABO blood group distribution was similar for the three Japanese cohorts — 29 to 30% Group O, 39 to 42% Group A, 20 to 21% Group B, and 9 to 10% Group AB — and different, as expected, from the distribution observed in caucasian populations. Hematocrit, serum glucose 1 hr after an oral 50 g glucose load, and uric acid values were similar in California and Hawaii and in both instances, higher than the values determined in Japan. Serum cholesterol values for the Hawaiian men were slightly lower than the values for the California Japanese men; both groups of migrants, however, had clearly higher serum cholesterol values than the native Japanese men — 217, 225, and 176 mg/dℓ, respectively.[66]

The calorie intake of the native Japanese was slightly lower than that of the Japanese men in Hawaii and California. The native Japanese consumed less protein (76 vs. 94 and 89 g), fat (36 vs. 85 and 95 g), and cholesterol (457 vs. 545 and 536 mg) but more total carbohydrate (335 vs. 260 and 251 g) and alcohol (28 vs. 13 and 9 g) than the migrant Japanese men living in Honolulu and California. The larger intakes of protein and fat observed in the two migrant groups result from greater intakes of animal protein and saturated animal fat; the larger intake of total carbohydrates in the cohort of native Japanese is related to larger intakes of complex carbohydrates, derived mainly from their high consumption of rice. The intake of simple carbohydrates, on the other hand, is greater among the two migrant groups of Japanese men.[66]

The protein intake contributes 14.3% of the calories in Japan, 16.7% in Hawaii, and 16.3% in California. The fat intake furnishes 15.1, 33.2, and 37.6% of the caloric intake observed among the native Japanese and the two migrant groups of Japanese men living in Honolulu and California, respectively. The 15% calorie contribution of dietary fat in Japan is well below the levels that have been suggested for intervention diets in areas with a high risk of developing CHD.[25,71] Dietary carbohydrate in Japan, Hawaii, and California provides 63.2, 46.4 and 44.1%, respectively, of the caloric intake of the study cohorts. The native Japanese derive 8.7% of their calories from alcoholic beverages, while in the two groups of Japanese-Americans, alcoholic beverages contribute 3.7% of the calories in Hawaii and 2.5% in California.[66]

Within a subclass of moderate smokers (less than one pack per day), the native Japanese men smoke more cigarettes than the Japanese living in either Honolulu or the San Francisco area in California. However, the proportion of heavy smokers (more than one pack per day), among native Japanese is similar to the proportion of heavy smokers among the Japanese men in California, and both rates are smaller than that observed among Japanese men in Honolulu.[66]

The baseline data comparisons described show differences between the native and migrant Japanese, particularly in terms of environmental and behavioral characteristics such as diet and cigarette smoking. Differences among the study cohorts are also apparent in attributes determined by a combination of genetic and environmental factors such as, for example, weight, serum cholesterol, and BP. On the other hand, only small differences are observed when the cohort populations are compared on the basis of characteristics that are primarily genetically determined such as blood type distribution, skeletal size, and height;[66] the latter, however, under certain conditions may be affected by nutritional factors, particularly during times of active growth and development.[72]

3. Diet and Atherosclerosis

Early results of autopsy studies in decedents from the population-based cohorts of Japanese men, residents of their native Japan and of Honolulu, Hawaii, indicate a more severe degree of aortic and coronary atherosclerosis in the Honolulu men,[5] based on estimates by the panel method proposed by the American Heart Association.[70]

Areas of myocardial necrosis and large myocardial scars were found more frequently in the deceased Japanese men who lived in Honolulu and both, severe atherosclerosis and myocardial lesions, were seen at younger ages in the Hawaii Japanese than in the native Japanese residents of Hiroshima.[5,34,73] Stemmermann and associates[5,73] attribute the apparent increase in severe ischemic lesions in the myocardium that they observe in the autopsied Hawaii Japanese to the earlier and more severe coronary atherosclerosis that these men had experienced.

Results of initial baseline examinations of the Honolulu Japanese also identify differences in the values of several biological and environmental parameters for these men when compared with corresponding values for Japanese men living in Japan and in California.[66] Since many of the parameters in reference can be considered potential risk factors for the development of CHD, Stemmermann and associates[73,74] used baseline information and autopsy findings available in the HHS to investigate atherosclerosis and its risk factors among Japanese men residents of Honolulu.

In the period between 1965 and 1974, 481 men who were participants in the HHS died. Autopsies were possible for 226 (47%) of the decedents and 137 (61%) of these autopsies were performed according to the standardized study protocol. The 137 decedents autopsied according to protocol were similar to the Japanese men in the total autopsy group who, in turn, were slightly younger and had a slightly lower systolic BP than the decedents that were not autopsied. The comparison of 11 additional decedent attributes by autopsy classification (protocol, routine, and no autopsy) did not suggest a serious bias in the selection of subjects for the protocol autopsies. Excluding the over representation of accidental deaths, frequently associated with population-based autopsy studies, the autopsied (protocol and routine) and nonautopsied decedents were similarly distributed with respect to four gross cause of death categories — CHD, stroke, cancer, and other or unknown.[34,73]

The associations of atherosclerosis grade with 16 to 20 antemortem factors, which included 4 to 9 dietary variables, were investigated at two successive points in time in the HHS by simple correlation analysis, simple regression and step-wise backward elimination multiple regression procedures.[34,73,74]

The simple correlation analysis in the first HHS exploration of associations of baseline data with degree of atherosclerosis in the aorta and the coronary arteries, included data available at the time for 124 and 109 decendents, respectively.[34,73] The results showed that age at death, systolic BP, and pulse were positive correlates of aortic atherosclerosis while vital capacity was inversely related to the aortic grade of atherosclerosis. Relative body weight, heart weight, serum cholesterol level, cigarettes smoked per day, 1-hr postprandial serum glucose, serum triglycerides, and hematocrit were identified by the correlation results as positive associates of coronary atherosclerosis, while the daily dietary intakes of calories and starch were negatively related to the coronary atherosclerosis grade.[34,73] The multivariate analysis results enhanced the apparent association of smoking with aortic atherosclerosis, but when the effect of concomitant variables is considered, the bivariate apparent associations of triglycerides, glucose, and hematocrit are no longer significant. It is not clear from these reports whether the dietary variables were or were not included in the multivariate analysis.[34,73]

The second HHS evaluation of associations of baseline data with aortic and coronary atherosclerosis included data available at the time for 178 and 165 decendents, respectively.[74] Results of the simple correlation analyses indicate that age at death, systolic BP, and serum cholesterol are strong positive associates of aortic atherosclerosis, while vital capacity again is identified as a strong negative associate of the atherosclerosis grade for the aorta; smoking and postprandial glucose are also directly related to the index of aortic atherosclerosis, while the dietary intake of carbohydrate

Table 3

SIMPLE CORRELATION COEFFICIENTS OF CORONARY AND
AORTIC GRADE OF ATHEROSCLEROSIS WITH SELECTED
ANTEMORTEM CHARACTERISTICS FROM TWO
SUBSEQUENT ANALYSIS OF DATA OF THE HONOLULU
HEART PROGRAM

Antemortem characteristic	First analysis[34,73]		Second analysis[74]	
	Coronaries[109]	Aorta[124]	Coronaries[165]	Aorta[178]
Systolic pressure (mmHg)	.14	.29	.17	.28
Serum cholesterol (mg/dl)	.35	.24	.30	.21
Relative weight (%)	.27	−.10	.18	−.03
Calorie intake (kcal/day)	−.23	−.10	−.22	−.13
Protein intake (g/day)	NR	NR	−.15	−.08
Fat intake (g/day)	NR	NR	−.09	−.10
Saturated fat intake (g/day)	−.11	−.09	−.09	−.10
Carbohydrate intake (g/day)	NR	NR	−.21	−.14
Sucrose intake (g/day)	NR	NR	−.06	−.10
Starch intake (g/day)	−.23	−.05	−.18	−.08
Cholesterol intake (mg/day)	NR	NR	−.02	−.04
Alcohol intake (g/day)	−.11	−.08	−.12	−.02

Figures in parenthesis specify the number of cases. NR = not reported.

appears to be inversely related to the index of atherosclerosis in the aorta. Serum cholesterol and postprandial glucose were identified as strong positive associates of coronary atherosclerosis while the daily intakes of calories and carbohydrates appeared as strong negative associates. The intake of starch is inversely related to coronary atherosclerosis, while relative weight, systolic BP, and age at death are positive associates of atherosclerosis in the coronary arteries.[74] The simultaneous consideration of variables by multivariate analyses rendered the bivariately observed associations of glucose and vital capacity with aortic atherosclerosis and those of age and glucose with coronary atherosclerosis nonsignificant. The association of cigarette smoking with atherosclerosis is enhanced in the multivariate analysis and becomes significant for both coronary and aortic atherosclerosis.[74]

The simple correlation coefficients of coronary and aortic atherosclerosis with systolic BP, serum cholesterol, relative weight, and the eight dietary variables considered in the analyses of the HHS data are presented in Table 3. The data included in this table identify serum cholesterol as the strongest and most consistent positive correlate of both aortic and coronary atherosclerosis, do not suggest an association of net dietary cholesterol with atherosclerosis in this autopsy sample and show uniformly negative correlations of dietary variables with the index of atherosclerosis. Many of these correlations, of course, are not different from zero.

4. Diet, Serum Lipids, and CHD

The baseline examinations provided 24-hr recall dietary information for over 7900 Japanese men in the HHS who also had laboratory results for serum cholesterol and serum triglyceride determinations on casual, nonfasting, blood samples. These results were used to explore associations of nutrient intake with serum lipids.[68] The baseline estimates of nutrient intake also provided an opportunity to investigate their relation to the observed incidence of CHD over cumulative time intervals.[69,76] The nutrients considered in these studies include calories, protein (animal and vegetable), fat (saturated, monounsaturated, and polyunsaturated fatty acids), carbohydrates (sugar, starch, and other carbohydrates), cholesterol, and alcohol. Simple linear regression, correlation and forward step-wise multiple regression procedures were used for the investigation of associations of nutrients and serum lipids.

The intakes of saturated fat, animal protein, and cholesterol, as well as the proportion of calories from total protein, animal protein, and saturated fat, were identified as contributors to higher serum cholesterol values by the simple linear regression analyses. On the other hand, the intakes of complex carbohydrates (starch) and of calories per unit of body weight, as well as the percent of calories from both complex and total carbohydrates, were inversely related to serum cholesterol values by the simple regression analyses. In all instances, however, the calculated correlation coefficients of nutrient intake with serum cholesterol were uniformly small, indicating that the associations identified are weak.[68]

The simple regression analyses revealed that there were few nutrients showing a significant relationship with serum triglycerides. However, the positive associations of saturated fat and simple carbohydrates in the diet with serum triglyceride levels, and the negative association of the dietary intake of complex carbohydrates with this serum lipid, according to Kato el al.[68] are consistent with current ideas but too weak for practical interpretation. The negative association of the intake of calories per unit of body weight with serum triglyceride levels is interpreted by the investigators as a reflection of the effect of calorie balance on triglycerides.

Percent calories from fat, calories per unit of body weight, total protein, simple carbohydrate, and total carbohydrate, in order of importance, were identified among the 17 dietary variables included in the step-wise regression analysis as the significant associates of serum cholesterol levels. The six variables combined, however, explained only 3.1% of the serum cholesterol variance, again indicating, at best, only a weak relation of nutrient intake and serum cholesterol. A similar analysis of data available for Japanese men, residents of Hiroshima and Nagasaki identified, in order of importance, the intakes of saturated fat, calories per unit of body weight, total calories, simple carbohydrate, percent calories from protein, animal protein, and cholesterol as diet variables which may be related to serum cholesterol values. In this analysis the seven dietary variables selected explained 8.5% of the serum cholesterol variance and although this is a little better than the corresponding result for the Japanese men in Hawaii, it still points only to a weak association. The inclusion of saturated fat and cholesterol among the selected dietary variables, however, is more in line with expectation.[68]

The inconsistency in the selection of variables in the two analyses and the small portion of serum cholesterol variance explained in both instances by the selected variables, suggest that other variables, dietary and nondietary, may relate more closely to serum cholesterol. Nevertheless, in both Hawaii and Japan, examination of nutrient intake by extreme quartiles in the distribution of serum cholesterol values showed that, in general, the men in the lower serum cholesterol quartile group had lower intakes of animal protein, saturated fat and dietary cholesterol. On the other hand, these men consumed more complex carbohydrates (starch) and had a more favorable calorie:weight ratio. The investigators interpret these results as an indication that it may be possible to lower serum lipid levels in a free living population by appropriate dietary changes.[68]

The estimates of the intake of nutrients for participants in the HHS were used to relate dietary variables to three groups of incidence of CHD and its manifestations during the 10 years subsequent to initial examination. The three groups of incidence are defined as follows: total CHD, myocardial infarction (MI) or CHD death, and angina (AP) or coronary insufficiency (CI). In case of multiple occurrences the subject was classified according to the more serious manifestation. The 18 nutrients considered in the analysis include: calories, protein, fat, saturated, monounsaturated, and polyunsaturated fatty acids, total, simple (sugar), complex (starch), and other carbohydrates, cholesterol, alcohol, percent calories from protein, fat, carbohydrates, and saturated fatty acids, and cholesterol per 1000 calories. Men who could not recall their food intake or indicated atypical intakes for the day of recall were excluded from the analyses. Also excluded were the men who at the time of initial examination were assessed as suffering latent CHD, stroke, or cancer. As a result, 918 men of the original 8006 with baseline data were excluded from the analyses.[75] Analysis of covariance was used to adjust for age differences and for testing differences in nutrient intake between a non-CHD group of men and the three groups of incidence defined above. The logistic model was used to test, in the presence of covariates, the relation of a particular dietary variate to disease outcome. The covariates used in these analyses include age, systolic BP, an index of physical activity, body weight, serum cholesterol, and cigarettes smoked.[75]

The 10-year incidence rate of fatal CHD and nonfatal MI observed in the cohort of Japanese men in the HHS is less than half the rate for white men in the U.S. and approximately double the rate for Japanese men in Japan.[76] The 456 men who developed CHD in this cohort during the 10-year reference period consumed fewer calories and had lower average daily intakes of carbohydrates, starch, and vegetable protein when compared with the men who did not develop CHD, MI, AP or CI during the time reference period. The men in the CHD groups obtained a greater portion of their average daily calories from protein, fat, saturated fatty acids, and polyunsaturated fatty acids than the men who remained healthy.[75]

The results of the multivariate analyses indicate that the net intakes of calories (−), starch (−), alcohol (−) and of cholesterol per 1000 calories (+), as well as the calorie contributions from protein (+) and fat (+) are significantly related to CHD. The results of these analyses, however, did not include either the intakes of carbohydrates and vegetable protein or the proportional calorie contributions from saturated and polyunsaturated fatty acids as significant associates of CHD.[75] Previous analyses by the group comparison approach of data available for the first 6 years of the HHS grossly identified the same relationships described for the 10-year data. However, when other major risk factors were taken into account in the multivariate logistic function analysis of the 6-year data, only the negative relations of alcohol and carbohydrate intake remained significant.[69]

In parallel with the studies of the relation of nutrient intake to CHD, the HHS information was used to explore the association of some biologic and lifestyle characteristics with the 10-year incidence of CHD.[76] In this case, the results of logistic multivariate analyses identified systolic BP as the most powerful and consistent risk factor for all manifestations of CHD with the exception of angina pectoris. Cigarette smoking showed a similar pattern, while serum cholesterol, although significantly related to fatal CHD and nonfatal MI, was not as strong a risk factor in the Hawaii cohort of Japanese men as either systolic BP or cigarette smoking.[76]

Viewed as a whole, the results of the HHS investigations of the relation of dietary variables with atherosclerosis, serum lipids, and CHD appear to be consistent in suggesting that the modification of diet may be a valuable instrument in efforts to lower serum lipids and retard atherosclerosis to reduce CHD morbidity and mortality.

IV. CLOSING REMARKS

The three studies we have reviewed in detail provide abundant information on the association of diet and diet-related factors with serum lipids, atherosclerosis, and some of the clinical manifestations of CHD. Of the three areas in reference, perhaps the one concerned with lesions has received least attention, probably because of the difficulties in obtaining dietary information for autopsied subjects without conducting an expensive prospective population-based cohort study. The autopsy study at present is practically the only way to obtain reliable estimates of atherosclerotic lesion involvement since quantitation of lesions in living subjects remains unreliable.[24] Autopsy studies also have well-recognized inherent limitations[24,30-33] that may condition the extension of results to the living population. The information on risk factor-lesion associations derived from the autopsy study (New Orleans) and the autopsy components of the two ongoing epidemiological prospective studies (Puerto Rico and Honolulu) considered in this review, clearly indicate their usefulness in the investigation of risk factors within the chain of events leading to the development of CHD.

The general agreement of the three studies in the identification of nutrition related risk factors is encouraging and suggests that the associations identified in common in the three studies may be real and not the result of chance. Gordon et al.,[77] while examining differences in CHD among Framingham, Honolulu, and Puerto Rico commented on the striking agreement among the studies with respect to the relationship of baseline characteristics to subsequent incidence of CHD. This suggests that agreement in findings is not limited to the studies reviewed but that it extends to other studies executed with different methodologies in widely different environments. Thus, Okumiya et al.,[6] as part of a prospective survey, graded atherosclerosis by the degree of luminal stenosis in 281 deceased persons over 40 years of age, residents of Hisayama, Japan. These investigators found a positive association of age, mean arterial BP, antemortem serum cholesterol, sex, and body mass index with coronary atherosclerosis. The seven variables selected by the multiple regression procedure used in the analysis explained 33.5% of the variance in coronary atherosclerosis. In the Oslo study, Holme et al.[78] found that serum cholesterol and BP were significant associates of coronary atherosclerosis, with serum cholesterol apparently more important than BP in the synergism affecting the development of coronary atherosclerosis; lesions in this case were quantitated using the IAP technique.[37,38] In the Framingham study, Feinleib and associates[79] used a clear plastic grid to map under ultraviolet (UV) light the areas of the intimal surface with lipid, complicated lesions and calcium deposits; the actual surface area was then carefully measured. They found a positive association of serum cholesterol with atherosclerotic involvement but no relation with BP by multiple regression analysis of 44 cases.

The apparent beneficial effects that can be expected from higher consumption of foods of vegetal origin and lower consumption of foods of animal origin, given the nutrient associations with serum lipids, lesion, and CHD identified by the comprehensive studies described in this review, agree with results obtained by other investigators under different circumstances and using different methods. Thus, recently Kahn et al.[80] studied the association between reported diet and all-cause mortality in a 21-year follow-up of 27,530 adult Seventh-Day Adventists in the U.S. Their results show that all-cause mortality was negatively related with the consumption of green salad and positively related with the consumption of eggs and meat. Kromhout and Coulander[81] investigated prevalence and mortality from CHD in a 10-year follow-up of 871 middle-aged men. Results of their analysis to examine diet-CHD associations show that dietary cholesterol per 1000 calories is positively and significantly related to CHD, while vegetable protein, polysacharides and dietary fiber are significantly and inversely related to CHD. The calorie intake per kilogram of body weight also was inversely related to CHD, but when subscapular skinfold and cholesterol were added to the logistic model used by these investigators, calories no longer appear related to CHD.

The results presented are consistent in suggesting that diet modifications designed to lower the intake of fat, particularly saturated fat, and to promote higher intakes of complex carbohydrates may have a beneficial effect in terms of lower serum cholesterol values, which in turn may lead to less atherosclerosis and eventually to a lower incidence of CHD. Although, the nutrient associations with serum lipids and atherosclerosis are generally weak and usually account for only a small amount of the variance of the dependent variables, the studies we have reviewed show that they are present at the three stages in the progression of the disease that were considered. However, even when diet changes can result in beneficial modifications of serum lipids as has been shown in clinical trials,[82] it is not clear if such changes may be induced in a free living population[83] given the difficulties associated with attempts to change lifestyles and particularly, dietary habits.

ACKNOWLEDGMENT

This work was supported in part by Grant HL-08974 from the National Heart, Lung and Blood Institute, National Institute of Health, U.S. Public Health Service, Bethesda, Md.

REFERENCES

1. White, P. D., Perspectives, *Progr. Cardiovasc. Dis.*, 14, 250, 1971.
2. Levy, R. I., Declining mortality in coronary heart disease, *Arteriosclerosis*, 1, 312, 1981.
3. Epstein, F. H., Coronary heart disease — geographical differences and time trends, in *Atherosclerosis VI*, Schettler, G., Gotto, A. M., Middelhoff, G., Habenicht, A. J. R., and Jurutka, K. R., Eds., Springer Verlag, New York, 1983, 723.
4. Stallones, R. A., The rise and fall of ischemic heart disease, *Sci. Am.*, 243, 53, 1980.
5. Stemmermann, G. N., Steer, A., Rhoads, G. G., Lee, K., Hayashi, T., Nakashima, T., and Keehn, R., A comparative pathology study of myocardial lesions and atherosclerosis in Japanese men living in Hiroshima, Japan and Honolulu, Hawaii, *Lab. Invest.*, 34, 592, 1976.
6. Okumiya, N., Tanaka, K., Ueda, K., and Omae, T., Coronary atherosclerosis and antecedent risk factors: pathologic and epidemiologic study in Hisayama, Japan, *Am. J. Cardiol.*, 56, 62, 1985.
7. WHO, *World Health Statistics Annual 1973-1976*, World Health Organization, Geneva, 1976.
8. Walker, W. J., Coronary mortality: what is going on?, *JAMA*, 227, 1045, 1974.
9. Gordon, T. and Thom, T., The recent decrease in CHD mortality, *Prevent. Med.*, 4, 115, 1975.
10. Lipid Research Clinics Program, The lipid research clinics coronary primary prevention trial results. I. Reduction in incidence of coronary heart disease, *JAMA*, 251, 351, 1984.
11. Ernst, N. D. and Levy, R. I., Diet and cardiovascular disease, in *Present Knowledge in Nutrition*, 5th ed., Olson, R. E., Broquist, H. P., Chichester, C. O., Darby, W. J., Kolbye, A. C., Jr., and Stalvey, R. M., Eds., The Nutrition Foundation, Washington, D.C., 1984, chap. 50.
12. Kimm, S. Y. S., Ornstein, S. M., DeLong, E. R., and Grufferman, S., Secular trends in ischemic heart disease mortality: regional variation, *Circulation*, 68, 3, 1983.
13. Strong, J. P., Solberg, L. A., and Restrepo, C., Atherosclerosis in persons with coronary heart disease, *Lab. Invest.*, 18, 527, 1968.
14. Deupree, R. H., Fields, R. I., McMahan, C. A., and Strong, J. P., Atherosclerotic lesions and coronary heart disease. Key relationships in necropsied cases, *Lab. Invest.*, 28, 252, 1973.
15. McGill, H. C., Jr., Introduction to the geographic pathology of atherosclerosis, *Lab. Invest.*, 18, 465, 1968.
16. Tejada, C., Strong, J. P., Montenegro, M. R., Restrepo, C., and Solberg, L. A., Distribution of coronary and aortic atherosclerosis by geographic location, race and sex, *Lab. Invest.*, 18, 509, 1968.
17. Strong, J. P. and Guzman, M. A., Decrease in coronary atherosclerosis in New Orleans, *Lab. Invest.*, 43, 297, 1980.
18. Strong, J. P. and McGill, H. C., Jr., The pediatric aspects of atherosclerosis, *J. Atherosclerosis Res.*, 9, 251, 1969.

19. Glueck, C. J., Laskarzewski, P. M., Morrison, J. A., Mellies, M. J., and Khoury, P. R., Pediatric precursors of atherosclerosis, in *Atherosclerosis VI,* Schettler, G., Gotto, A. M., Middelhoff, G., Habenicht, A. J. R., and Jurutka, K. R., Eds., Springer-Verlag, New York, 1983, 745.
20. Holman, R. L., McGill, H. C., Jr., Strong, J. P., and Geer, G. C., The natural history of atherosclerosis. The early aortic lesions as seen in New Orleans in the middle of the 20th century, *Am. J. Pathol.,* 34, 209, 1958.
21. Oalmann, M. C., Palmer, R. W., Guzman, M. A., and Strong, J. P., Sudden death coronary heart disease, atherosclerosis and myocardial lesions in young men, *Am. J. Epidemiol.,* 112, 639, 1980.
22. Berkson, D. M. and Stamler, J., Epidemiology of the killer chronic diseases, in *Nutrition and the Killer Diseases,* Winick, M., Ed., John Wiley & Sons, New York, 1981, 17.
23. Kannel, W. B., McGee, D., and Gordon, T., A general cardiovascular risk profile: the Framingham study, *Am. J. Cardiol.,* 38, 46, 1976.
24. Solberg, L. A. and Strong, J. P., Risk factors and atherosclerotic lesions. A review of autopsy studies, *Arteriosclerosis,* 3, 187, 1983.
25. National Institutes of Health Consensus Development Panel, Lowering blood cholesterol to prevent heart disease. NIH Consensus Development Conference statement, *Arteriosclerosis,* 5, 404, 1985.
26. Bronte-Stewart, B., Keys, A., and Brock, J. F., Serum-cholesterol, diet and coronary heart disease, *Lancet,* 2, 1103, 1955.
27. Keys, A., *Seven Countries: A Multivariate Analysis of Death and Coronary Heart Disease,* Harvard University Press, Cambridge, 1980.
28. Malmros, H., The relation of nutrition to health: a statistical study of the effect of the war-time on arteriosclerosis, cardiosclerosis, tuberculosis and diabetes, *Acta Med. Scand.,* (Suppl. 246), 137, 1950.
29. Ström, A. and Jensen, R. A., Mortality from circulatory diseases in Norway 1940 to 1945, *Lancet,* 1, 126, 1951.
30. Guzman, M. A., Correlation of the nutritional and pathological aspects of cardiovascular disease, in *Nutrition in Health and Disease and International Development: Symposia From the XII International Congress of Nutrition,* Harper, A. E. and Davis, G. K., Eds., Alan R. Liss, New York, 1981, 821.
31. McMahan, C. A., Autopsied cases by age, sex and "race", *Lab. Invest.,* 18, 8, 1968.
32. Carlson, H. A. and Bell, E. T., Statistical study of occurrence of cancer and tuberculosis in 11,195 post-mortem examinations, *J. Cancer Res.,* 13, 126, 1929.
33. Mainland, D., The risk of fallacious conclusions from autopsy data on the incidence of diseases with applications to heart diseases, *Am. Heart J.,* 45, 644, 1953.
34. Rhoads, G. G., Blackwelder, W. C., Stemmermann, G. N., Hayashi, T., and Kagan, A., Coronary risk factors and autopsy findings in Japanese-American men, *Lab. Invest.,* 38, 304, 1978.
35. Sorlie, P. D., Garcia-Palmieri, M. R., Castillo-Staab, M. I., Costas, R., Jr., Oalmann, M. C., and Havlick, R., The relation of antemortem factors to atherosclerosis at autopsy. The Puerto Rico Heart Health Program, *Am. J. Pathol.,* 103, 345, 1981.
36. Stamler, J., Population studies, in *Nutrition, Lipids and Coronary Heart Disease — A Global View,* Levy, R., Rifkind, B., Dennis, B., and Ernst, N. D., Eds., Raven Press, New York, 1979, 25.
37. Guzman, M. A., McMahan, C. A., McGill, H. C., Jr., Strong, J. P., Tejada, C., Restrepo, C., Eggen, D. A., Robertson, W. B., and Solberg, L. A., Selected methodologic aspects of the International Atherosclerosis Project, *Lab. Invest.,* 18, 479, 1968.
38. Guzman, M. A., McMahan, C. A., and Strong, J. P., Unaided visual estimation of atherosclerotic lesions: biological variability compared with grading variability, *Lab. Invest.,* 31, 398, 1974.
39. Interamerican Atherosclerosis Project, Standard Operating Protocol, Department of Pathology, Louisiana State University and Instituto de Nutricion de Centro America y Panama, Guatemala, 1962.
40. Scrimshaw, N. S. and Guzman, M. A., Diet and atherosclerosis, *Lab. Invest.,* 18, 623, 1968.
41. Strong, J. P., Richards, M. L., McGill, H. C., Jr., Eggen, D. A., and McMurry, M. T., On the association of cigarette smoking with coronary and aortic atherosclerosis, *J. Atheroscler. Res.,* 10, 303, 1969.
42. Strong, J. P. and Richards, M. L., Cigarette smoking and atherosclerosis in autopsied men, *Atherosclerosis,* 23, 451, 1976.
43. Moore, M. C., Moore, E. M., Beasley, C. deH., Hankins, G. J., and Judlin, B. C., Dietary atherosclerosis study on deceased persons: methodology, *Am. J. Dietet. Assoc.,* 56, 13, 1970.
44. Moore, M. C., Judlin, B. C. and Kennemur, P. McA., Using graduated food models in taking dietary histories, *J. Am. Dietet. Assoc.,* 51, 447, 1967.
45. Moore, M. C., *Extended Table of Nutrient Values,* International Dietary Information Foundation, Atlanta, 1974.

46. Moore, M. C., Guzman, M. A., Schilling, P. E., and Strong, J. P., Dietary-atherosclerosis study on deceased persons: relation of eating pattern to raised coronary lesions, *J. Am. Dietet. Assoc.,* 67, 22, 1975.

47. Moore, M. C., Guzman, M. A., Schilling, P. E., and Strong, J. P., Dietary-atherosclerosis study on deceased persons: relation of selected dietary components to raised coronary lesions, *J. Am. Dietet. Assoc.,* 68, 216, 1976.

48. Jick, H., Miettinen, O. S., Neff, R. K., Shapiro, S., Heinonen, O. P., and Slone, D., Coffee and myocardial infarction, *N. Engl. J. Med.,* 289, 63, 1973.

49. Hennekens, C. H., Drolette, M. E., Jesse, M. J., Davies, J. E., and Hutchison, G. B., Coffee drinking and death due to coronary heart disease, *N. Engl. J. Med.,* 294, 633, 1976.

50. Yano, K., Rhoads, G. G., and Kagan, A., Coffee, alcohol, and risk of CHD among Japanese men living in Hawaii, *N. Engl. J. Med.,* 297, 405, 1977.

51. Bray, G. A., Lipogenesis in human adipose tissue — some effects of nibbling and gorging, *J. Clin. Invest.,* 51, 537, 1972.

52. Metzner, H. L., Lamphiear, D. E., Wheeler, M. C., and Larkin, F. A., The relationship between frequency of eating and adiposity in adult men and women in the Tecumseh Community Health Study, *Am. J. Clin. Nutr.,* 30, 712, 1977.

53. Strong, J. P., An introduction to the epidemiology of atherosclerosis, in *Atherosclerosis IV,* Schettler, G., Goto, Y., Hata, Y., and Klose, G., Eds., Springer Verlag, New York, 1977, 92.

54. Ernst, N., and Levy, R. I., Diet, hyperlipidemia and atherosclerosis, in *Modern Nutrition in Health and Disease,* 6th ed., Lea and Febiger, Philadelphia, 1980, 1045.

55. Moore, M. C., Guzman, M. A., Schilling, P. E., and Strong, J. P., Dietary-atherosclerosis study on deceased persons: further data on the relation of selected nutrients to raised coronary lesions, *J. Am. Dietet. Assoc.,* 70, 601, 1977.

56. Grande, F., Anderson, J. T., and Keys, A., Sucrose and various carbohydrate containing foods and serum lipids in man, *Am. J. Clin. Nutr.,* 27, 1043, 1974.

57. Garcia-Palmieri, M. R., Sorlie, P., Tillotson, J., Costas, R., Jr., Cordero, E., and Rodriguez, M., Relationship of dietary intake to subsequent coronary heart disease incidence: the Puerto Rico Heart Health Program, *Am. J. Clin. Nutr.,* 33, 1818, 1980.

58. Carroll, K. K., Dietary proteins and amino acids — their effects on cholesterol metabolism, in *Animal and Vegetable Proteins in Lipid Metabolism and Atherosclerosis,* Gibney, M. J. and Kritchevsky, D., Eds., Alan R. Liss, New York, 1983, 9.

59. Kritchevsky, D., Tepper, S. A., Czarnecki, S. K., Klurfeld, D. M., and Story, J. A., Effects of Animal and vegetable protein in experimental atherosclerosis, in *Animal and Vegetable Proteins in Lipid Metabolism and Atherosclerosis,* Gibney, M. J. and Kritchevsky, D., Eds., Alan R. Liss, New York, 1983, 85.

60. Bressani, R. and Navarrete, D. A., Niacin content of coffee in Central America, *Food Res.,* 24, 344, 1959.

61. Hegsted, D. M., McGandy, R. B., Myers, M. L., and Stare, F. J., Quantitative effects of dietary fat on serum cholesterol in man, *Am. J. Clin. Nutr.,* 17, 281, 1965.

62. Moore, M. C., Guzman, M. A., Schilling, P. E., and Strong, J. P., Dietary-atherosclerosis study on deceased persons: relation of certain market foods to raised coronary lesions, *J. Am. Dietet. Assoc.,* 79, 668, 1981.

63. Garcia-Palmieri, M. R., Feliberti, M., Costas, R., Jr., Colon, A. A., Cruz-Vidal, M., Cortez-Alicea, M., Ayala, A. M., Sobrino, R., and Torres, R., An epidemiological study on coronary heart disease in Puerto Rico: the Puerto Rico Heart Health Program, *Bol. Asoc. Med. P.R.,* 61, 174, 1969.

64. Garcia-Palmieri, M. R., Castillo, M. I., Oalmann, M. C., Sorlie, P. D., and Costas, R., Jr., The relation of ante mortem factors to atherosclerosis at necropsy, in *Atherosclerosis IV,* Schettler, G., Goto, Y., Hata, Y., and Klose, G., Eds., Springer Verlag, New York, 1977, 108.

65. Garcia-Palmieri, M. R., Tillotson, J., Cordero, E., Costas, R., Jr., Sorlie, P., Gordon, T., Kannel, W. B., and Colon, A. A., Nutrient intake and serum lipids in urban and rural Puerto Rican men, *Am. J. Clin. Nutr.,* 30, 2092, 1977.

66. Kagan, A., Harris, B. R., Winkelstein, W., Jr., Johnson, K. G., Kato, H., Syme, S. L., Rhoads, G. G., Gay, M. L., Nichaman, M. Z., Hamilton, H. B., and Tillotson, J., Epidemiologic studies of coronary heart disease and stroke in Japanese men living in Japan, Hawaii and California: demographic, physical, dietary and biochemical characteristics, *J. Chron. Dis.,* 27, 345, 1974.

67. Tillotson, J., Kato, H., Nichaman, M. Z., Miller, D. C., Gay, M. L., Johnson, K. G., and Rhoads, G. G., Epidemiology of coronary heart disease and stroke in Japanese men living in Japan, Hawaii and California: methodology for comparison of diet, *Am. J. Clin. Nutr.,* 26, 177, 1973.

68. Kato, H., Tillotson, J., Nichaman, M. Z., Rhoads, G. G., and Hamilton, H. B., Epidemiologic studies of coronary heart disease and stroke in Japanese men living in Japan, Hawaii and California: serum lipids and diet, *Am. J. Epidemiol.,* 97, 372, 1973.

69. Yano, K., Rhoads, G. G., Kagan, A., and Tillotson, J., Dietary intake and the risk of coronary heart disease in Japanese men living in Hawaii, *Am. J. Clin. Nutr.*, 31, 1270, 1978.

70. McGill, H. C., Jr., Brown, B. W., Gore, I., McMillan, G. C., Paterson, J. C., Pollak, O. J., Roberts, J. C., and Wissler, R. W., Grading human atherosclerotic lesions using a panel of photographs, *Circulation*, 37, 455, 1968.

71. Rinzler, S. H., Primary prevention of coronary heart disease by diet, *Bull. N.Y. Acad. Med.*, 44, 936, 1968.

72. Guzman, M. A., Impaired physical growth and maturation in malnourished populations, in *Malnutrition, Learning and Behavior*, Scrimshaw, N. S. and Gordon, J. E., Eds., M.I.T. Press, Cambridge, Mass., 1968, 42.

73. Stemmermann, G. N., Rhoads, G. G., and Blackwelder, W. C., Atherosclerosis and its risk factors in the Hawaiian Japanese, in *Atherosclerosis IV*, Schettler, G., Goto, Y., Hata, Y., and Klose, G., Eds., Springer Verlag, New York, 1977, 113.

74. Stemmermann, G. N., Rhoads, G. G., and Hayashi, T., Atherosclerosis and its risk factors among Hawaii Japanese, in *Atherosclerosis V*, Gotto, A. M., Jr., Smith, L. C., and Allen, B., Eds., Springer Verlag, New York, 1980, 63.

75. McGee, D. L., Reed, D. M., Yano, K., Kagan, A., and Tillotson, J., Ten-year incidence of coronary heart disease in the Honolulu Heart Program: relationship to nutrient intake, *Am. J. Epidemiol.*, 119, 667, 1984.

76. Yano, K., Reed, D. M., and McGee, D. L., Ten-year incidence of coronary heart disease in the Honolulu Heart Program: relationship to biologic and lifestyle characteristics, *Am. J. Epidemiol.*, 119, 653, 1984.

77. Gordon, T., Garcia-Palmieri, M. R., Kagan, A., Kannel, W. B., and Schiffman, J., Differences in coronary heart disease in Framingham, Honolulu and Puerto Rico, *J. Chron. Dis.*, 27, 329, 1974.

78. Holme, I., Enger, S. C., Helgeland, I. H., Leren, P., Lund-Larsen, P. G., Solberg, L. A., and Strong, J. P., Risk factors and raised atherosclerotic lesions in coronary and cerebral arteries, *Arteriosclerosis*, 1, 250, 1981.

79. Feinlab, M., Kannel, W. B., Tedeschi, C. G., Landau, T. K., and Garrison, R. J., The relation of antemortem characteristics to cardiovascular findings at necropsy, *Atherosclerosis*, 34, 145, 1979.

80. Kahn, H. A., Phillips, R. L., Snowdon, D. A., and Choi, W., Association between reported diet and all-cause mortality: twenty-one-year follow-up on 27530 adult seventh-day adventists, *Am. J. Epidemiol.*, 119, 775, 1984.

81. Kromhout, D. and Coulander, Cor DeLezenne, Diet, prevalance and 10-year mortality from coronary heart disease in 871 middle-aged men: the Zutphen Study, *Am. J. Epidemiol.*, 119, 733, 1984.

82. Ahrens, E. H., Jr., Blankenhorn, D. H., and Tsaltas, T. T., Effect on human serum lipids of substituting plant for animal fat in the diet, *Proc. Soc. Exp. Biol. Med.*, 86, 872, 1954.

83. Goldberg, S. J., Allen, H. D., Friedman, G., Meredith, K., Tymrack, M., and Owen, A. Y., Use of health education and attempted dietary change to modify atherosclerotic risk factors: a controlled trial, *Am. J. Clin. Nutr.*, 33, 1272, 1980.

INDEX